The Healing Art of
SPORTS
MASSAGE

The Healing Art of
SPORTS
MASSAGE

By Joan Johnson

Director, Sports Massage of the Rockies

Rodale Press, Inc.
Emmaus, Pennsylvania

Cover and Book Designer: Charles Beasley
Cover Photographer: Mitch Mandel

Library of Congress Cataloging-in-Publication Data

Johnson, Joan.
    The healing art of sports massage / Joan Johnson.
        p.   cm.
      Includes index.
      ISBN 0–87596–186–X   paperback
      1. Massage.   2. Sports physical therapy.   I. Title.
RC1226.J64   1995
615.8′22—dc20   94-45679

Distributed in the book trade by St. Martin's Press

2 4 6 8 10 9 7 5 3 1 paperback

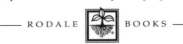

OUR MISSION
We publish books that empower people's lives.
RODALE BOOKS

To Myron Wood and a friend, Michelle Conrad,
and my two writing companions, my cats

CONTENTS

ACKNOWLEDGMENTS . . . . *viii*

FOREWORD . . . . *ix*

INTRODUCTION . . . . *x*

CHAPTER 1 THE ROOTS OF SPORTS MASSAGE *1*

CHAPTER 2 PREPARING YOUR HANDS *7*

CHAPTER 3 TOOLS OF THE TRADE *13*

CHAPTER 4 MASSAGE TECHNIQUES MADE EASY . .*25*

CHAPTER 5 SELF-MASSAGE TECHNIQUES *75*

CHAPTER 6 SPORT-SPECIFIC MASSAGES *91*

CHAPTER 7 RECOVERY FROM HARD EFFORTS . .*127*

CHAPTER 8 STAYING FREE OF INJURY *135*

CHAPTER 9 MASSAGE FOR THE MIND *143*

CHAPTER 10 WHAT THE ATHLETES SAY *151*

INDEX *159*

ACKNOWLEDGMENTS

This book would not be possible without the influence of many people. These include:

Sally Edwards, Bart Yasso and Don Kardong, who suggested this book.

Publisher Pat Corpora, managing editor Sharon Faelten and editor Sara Henry of Rodale Press, who were my coaches throughout the creation of this book, and Cate Terwilliger and John Teaford, who lent valuable writing assistance.

Arturo Barrios, Mark Plaatjes, Nadia Prasad, Kim Jones, Mike Pigg and numerous other athletes—particularly in the community of Boulder, Colorado—who have taught me much about body, mind and spirit.

My fellow massage therapists, who have one of the most humanistic and compassionate occupations in the world, and the American Massage Therapy Association, which has given our profession attention, respect and acknowledgment. Special thanks to Kevin Belden, University of Colorado athletics department massage therapist, for serving as the model for some of the illustrations.

Bob and Jean Anderson, author and illustrator, respectively, of *Stretching* and an enormous inspiration for me; Jane Hall, my high school Latin teacher, for giving me the love of language; and T. C. Valentine, for his sports psychology theories.

My teachers in sports science at Iowa State University; the folks at the Olympic Training Center in Colorado Springs; and my friends at the *Washington Post*.

And, finally, my brother David, who piqued my interest in massage when I was 15 by giving me a copy of *The Massage Book* by George Downing; also, my other siblings and especially my mother and father, who have given me love, support and inspiration along the way.

FOREWORD

When I started running in Johannesburg, South Africa, massage was not a weekly or even a monthly ritual for me. When my legs hurt after a hard training session or a race, I would rub analgesic on the sore areas. Sometimes I would just take a few days off until my legs felt better. As I learned more about physiology and anatomy and trained more intensely, I realized that if I rubbed my legs well before and after hard efforts and races, I recovered much more quickly.

In physical therapy school, I learned more complicated massage techniques, and I started practicing on people. All the while, however, I never quite followed through by using these principles and techniques to aid my own running. It was not until I moved to Boulder, Colorado, that I truly realized the importance of regular massage. In Boulder I met many athletes who were running professionally and making a good living from their talents. I realized that besides training hard, eating well and allowing adequate time for rest and recovery, all these athletes had a thorough massage at least once a week.

When we train hard or race, we repeatedly subject our muscles to microtrauma. The body heals microtrauma to tendons, muscles and ligaments by generating more collagen, a connective-tissue protein that your body uses as a "cement." Massage aids the healing process and hastens recovery by breaking up excess collagen materials between healthy muscle fibers, increasing circulation, flushing out lactic acid and other toxins and helping maintain muscle length.

For the past four years, Joan Johnson, together with my physical therapy support crew, has kept me healthy and injury-free. Joan has developed a wonderful repertoire of massage techniques, along with a unique sensitivity and knowledge of each of her client's muscles, that keeps her schedule filled. Those of us who go to Joan for massages regularly realize the integral role she plays in our progress while training and racing. I'm delighted that Joan has decided to share her techniques in book form, where it can reach so many who will enjoy the multiple benefits of the art of massage.

—*Mark Plaatjes, registered physical therapist, RPT Associates, Boulder, Colorado, and 1993 World Marathon champion*

INTRODUCTION

I wrote this book to share my experience of more than a decade in private practice as a sports massage therapist and to convey the message that I've learned alongside my clients: Sports massage is one of the best, most effective ways to help people help themselves. Among other benefits, it can help prevent injuries, hasten recovery from hard workouts and injuries and help you relax.

I've been blessed with a client list that includes Mark Allen, Arturo Barrios, Colleen Cannon, Gwyn Coogan, Wes Hobson, Paula Newby-Fraser, Mike Pigg, Mark Plaatjes, Nadia Prasad, Frank Shorter, Ken Souza, Scott Tinley, Jill Trenary, Craig Virgin and many other world-class and Olympic athletes. After starting my private practice on the sports circuit while cross-training as a competitive athlete, I lived for six years in Colorado Springs, where I worked with local athletes and those at the U.S. Olympic Training Center. I now live in Boulder—a mecca not only for athletes but also for outstanding mind/body therapists—and here I operate Sports Massage of the Rockies.

The Healing Art of Sports Massage will allow you to explore the basic components of massage by giving you a simple and basic structure that you can follow and use as a springboard for your own creativity. The book's illustrations and design have been planned to make learning as user-friendly as possible. Leave it open at your side while trying some of the techniques on a friend or during self-massage.

This book contains most of the practical information that you will want to explore before beginning. If you've never done massage before, don't worry. Like sports themselves, massage is so natural that everyone is capable of it. I believe everyone is a natural athlete; therefore, everyone is a natural massage therapist.

Start small—there is an ever-evolving learning process in this healing art. Whenever you can, have the strokes done on you. And don't be intimidated by what may seem to be complex movements—the strokes are much easier than they may appear on paper.

Massage makes us feel more whole. It is a gift that your hands have the power to give to yourself and to your friends. Learn to give and receive. Learn to trust this gift, and you will experience what massage is all about.

—*Joan Johnson*

1

THE ROOTS OF SPORTS MASSAGE

In the evolution of the senses, the sense of touch was undoubtedly the first to come into being."

ASHLEY MONTAGU, *Touching: The Human Significance of Skin*

Whether you're a weekend warrior, a professional athlete or an active individual who works hard to stay fit, sports massage can do far more than provide a feeling of pleasure or relief for the overworked body—it can rejuvenate body, mind and spirit.

One of the many people I massage is Arturo Barrios, who held the world record in the 10,000 meters for nearly four years. Arturo has massages twice a week, after each of his intense track workouts. Each of these 60- to 90-minute sessions gives his muscles the chance to begin to relax. But massage also helps identify irregularities that could turn into problems if not treated or allowed to recover. Sports massage has kept Arturo remarkably injury-free and has speeded his recovery from hard workouts.

"Whenever I race, it used to take me two or three days to recover," says

Arturo. "But if I get a massage the day after, it only takes a few hours to feel back on track and ready for another demanding workout."

WHAT SPORTS MASSAGE CAN DO FOR YOU

Athletes around the world and at all levels of ability and accomplishment now rely on massage as an indispensable part of their training programs. Studies in the United States, Australia and the former Soviet Union have shown that sports massage techniques, when used regularly as part of a regimented training program, increase the blood flow that is vital to recovery, improve the range of motion and strength of injured muscles and accelerate gains in muscle strength.

HOW SPORTS MASSAGE HELPS YOU

What is the difference between regular massage and sports massage? Basically, non-sports massage is more superficial and does not target specific muscle groups that are used in sports activity.

In sports massage, the techniques are designed to benefit muscles by warming and softening tissue, realigning muscle fibers, helping to heal scar tissue and flushing toxins from specific muscles. A regular massage may relax you and make you feel great, but it won't specifically benefit the muscles or body parts that you've stressed in your workout.

In summary, regular sports massage can:

- Help identify tender areas before they develop into injuries
- Enhance overall body awareness
- Stretch and relax muscles
- Relieve muscle pain and spasms
- Free muscle adhesions and soften scar tissue caused by injury
- Improve range of motion
- Restore suppleness and elasticity
- Improve circulation of blood and lymph fluids
- Flush out toxins that cause muscle stiffness and soreness
- Speed recovery from muscular exertion
- Relax the mind and body

Overuse injuries are a fact. Regular sports massage restores the length and suppleness of muscles that become tight and tense from physical exertion. Additionally, microtears in the muscles from training heal faster because massage aids circulation of blood and nutrients and enables the body to adapt to increased workloads. And long before an injury becomes painful, the probing required in sports massage may help detect stress areas before they become chronic problems. In short, sports massage keeps muscles healthy and flexible, so tears and strains are less likely.

Any athlete who cross-trains knows that increased workouts lead to improved performance. But some neglect an equally important area—recovery. With a full recovery, you will be able to push previous boundaries and adapt to a new level of stress. Why carry your soreness and stiffness from your last workout with you? Why not take measures now to speed your recovery from your effort so you can reach a higher level in your next workout? Sports massage provides the secret weapon for complete recovery.

Finally, nothing is more essential to positive change than self-esteem, self-awareness and self-confidence. Massage is a direct way to increase total body awareness—and it feels great.

HOW MASSAGE GOT STARTED

Touch, the mother of our senses, is the core of massage. It is the sense that Diane Ackerman, in her wonderful book *The Natural History of the Senses*, describes as the "oldest . . . and the most urgent." Indeed, this primal sense and the word *massage* itself are inseparable—its French root, *masser*, has its origins in the Arabic word *massa*, which means "to touch."

The idea that touch can have a direct, significant, therapeutic value is far from new, as Patricia J. Benjamin points out in an article in the American Massage Therapy Association's *Massage Journal*. Massage is mentioned in the earliest documentation in China, *The Yellow Emperor's Classic of Internal Medicine*, circa 2598 B.C. In the eleventh century B.C., the Arab philosopher-physician Avicenna noted in his writings that massage could "disperse the effect matters found in the muscles and not expelled by exercise." Sanskrit texts carved into the temples of India contain reliefs of Buddha receiving massage treatments.

The Greeks and Romans popularized massage—physicians recommended it as part of a health care regimen that included exercise and mineral baths, and Homer's *Odyssey* mentions it as a welcome relief for exhausted heroes. Hippocrates, the Greek physician commonly associated with the founding of physical medicine, found massage a vital principle in therapeutic modalities, insisting that it be made part of physical training. "The physician must be experienced in many things," he said, "but most assuredly in rubbing . . . for rubbing can bind a joint that is too loose and loosen a joint that is too rigid."

Plutarch tells us in his writings that Julius Caesar used massage for his epilepsy and for recovery from his prodigious labors. And Pliny the Elder, the great Roman naturalist, had himself rubbed as part of his daily baths for relief from asthma.

From the Middle Ages until the sixteenth century, massage found little encouragement in Europe amid widespread taboos concerning pleasures of the flesh. In the East, however, massage, acupuncture, acupressure and shiatsu (a blend of massage and acupressure) were much valued for their healing properties. East finally began to meet West in the 1800s, largely due to the efforts of a Swede named Per Henrick Ling.

Ling, born in 1776, practiced and taught the style of massage most familiar today and now known as Swedish massage. As the nineteenth century dawned, Ling expanded upon the techniques of the Orient as they were translated into French, devising a systematic approach to holistic health. This program, like its Greek and Roman predecessors, went beyond massage, advocating the consumption of mineral waters, as well as taking regular mineral baths and following graduated exercise programs. Ling, a fencing master and instructor of gymnastics and movement, based his system on physiology. As his methods won acceptance in Europe, institutes based on this system—called the Swedish Movement Treatment—sprang up in Germany, Austria and France. The Swedish government included his system in the nation's schools, and today the American Massage Therapy Association (AMTA) considers it the blueprint for creating standards in massage.

THE PROFESSION GAINS RESPECT

Between 1854 and 1920 the practice of massage developed further. Once a relatively unskilled labor, massage began to assume a place among other health care services as a few prominent physicians educated at Ling's Central Institute in Stockholm struck a balance among drugs, surgery and more natural healing methods. In 1860, George H. Taylor, M.D., wrote of the Ling system in a book called *Health by Exercise,* and opened institutes in New York based on those in Europe.

John G. Trine, M.D., brought the system west to Chicago. John H. Kellogg, M.D., the well-known health crusader from Battle Creek, Michigan, employed masseuses and masseurs and in 1895 published the popular book *The Art of Massage.* Other works followed as Swedes who were educated in their homeland's institutes emigrated to the United States. Many massage texts were translated into English, including Kurre Ostrom's *Massage and the Original Swedish Movements*, published in 1890. By the 1920s, R. Tait McKenzie, a physician and physical educator, held a full-time professorship in physical therapy and insisted that massage be taught in conjunction with anatomy and physiology.

Unfortunately, McKenzie's was a voice in the wilderness. While hands-on therapies flourished in Europe and Asia, they were incompatible with cultural norms then prevalent in America. (Later, in the 1960s and 1970s, "massage parlors" sprang up nationwide, but these had more to do with selling sex than with soothing over-taxed muscles.) And while the development of medical theory and practice took major strides in the nineteenth and twentieth centuries, the practice of hands-on treatments declined steadily. In 1943, a group of massage therapists founded the American Association of Masseurs and Masseuses, now known as the American Massage Therapy Association (AMTA). Nevertheless, new therapeutic technologies such as ultrasound began to supplant the time-consuming art of massage, and manual massage drifted out of the medical mainstream and into vacation resorts, health clubs and beauty salons.

A Welcome Trend

Today, the pendulum is beginning to reverse its swing. Sports medicine literature from eastern Europe and the former Soviet Union contains a wealth of scientific studies citing the benefits of massage. Top American athletes (such as Tour de France winner Greg LeMond, Olympic gold medalist swimmer Janet Evans, track and field star Jackie Joyner-Kersee and many, many more) have discovered for them-selves its preventive and restorative value.

As the number of Americans taking part in competitive events has grown, so has the visibility of the massage therapist, who often can be seen tending to a long line of weary runners or cyclists after a weekend event. Indeed, one factor behind the increasing demand for therapeutic and sports massage may be the trend toward self-responsibility in health care—keeping the body well through exercise, diet, relaxation and stress reduction.

The basic philosophies of traditional and alternative therapies and health care have been divided by miles of mistrust and misunderstanding, but massage for athletes is helping to bridge the gap as alternative and holistic methods again find a place in sports medicine. Nowhere else is the adage "an ounce of prevention is worth a pound of cure" more appropriate. Sports care grew out of the need for ways to heal injured athletes without a complete cessation of training and, where possible, without surgery or drugs. By using the preventive powers of massage, we can detect problems before they become chronic and, best of all, keep injuries at a minimum.

Since the 1980s, massage therapy has rapidly developed into a new profes-sion. The AMTA works toward establishing credibility through legislation and structuring massage therapy as an occupation on an equal footing with others in our health care system, as it was in Hippocrates' day.

History is beginning to repeat itself.

CHAPTER

2

PREPARING YOUR HANDS

No single therapeutic agent can be compared in efficiency with this
familiar but perfect tool . . . the human hand. If half as much
research had been expended on the principles governing manual
treatment as upon pharmacology, the hand would be esteemed today
on a par with drugs in acceptability and power.

J. MADISON TAYLOR, M.D.

Don't your hands get tired?" is a question I hear frequently. The answer is "Of course." But learning to be at one with your technique and style helps. Although it has taken me years to reach this level of endurance, usually I can do up to six full-body sessions of an hour and a half each before I need to take a break. I think of it as running several marathons—with my hands.

The best way to build specific power for massage is, of course, through the practice of massage. You can, however, accelerate your hands' development through some simple exercises. You can strengthen your fingers by using foam or metal hand grippers, which you can find at sporting goods stores, or by simply squeezing a chunk of clay or a tennis ball.

Once or twice a day, say while you're reading or watching television, grip the ball or clay, first with your entire hand and then with your thumb and each individual finger. Squeeze until your hand becomes tired. After a workout, stretch your hands, separating and extending the fingers as shown. This basic strength workout, which you can incorporate into your daily routine until it becomes almost subconscious, will safely and gradually build power in the hands, wrists and forearms. These strengthening exercises will help prevent injuries, too.

▼ After working out your fingers, stretch as shown for 10 seconds, then make a tight fist and hold for 10 seconds, then bend your knuckles for another 10 seconds. Repeat several times.

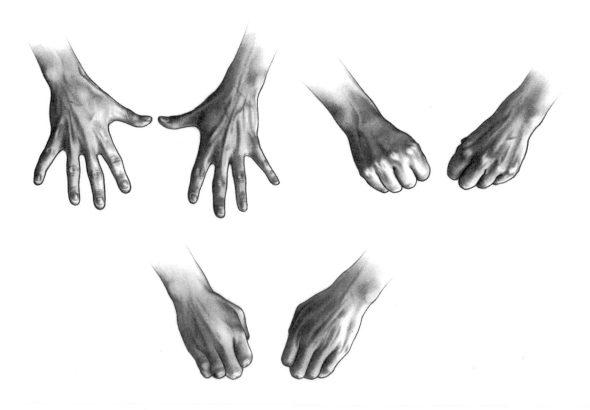

If you want to strengthen your fingers more, consider buying a training device common to rock climbers—the finger board, which has a number of different-size holds to hang from. You can find a selection of boards at your local outdoor or mountaineering shop for $45 and up. Warm up your hands, wrists and forearms first by starting on the largest rounded holds and hanging, relaxed, for 5 to 10 seconds. This strengthens both your hands and forearms. Move slowly around the board, alternating from large to small holds. Use the finger board when your hands are fresh (not after giving a massage or after weight lifting, for example); take your time and don't overexert yourself.

Here's a sample workout that you can try.

- Small hold: Hang for 7 seconds; rest for 60 seconds. Repeat up to three times.

- Medium hold: Hang for 12 seconds; rest for 60 seconds. Repeat twice.

- Large hold: Hang for 20 seconds; rest for 60 seconds. Then hang for 12 seconds; rest for 60 seconds. Repeat once.

- Small hold: Hang for 7 seconds.

By the workout's end, your muscles should be fatigued. Don't forget to gently stretch your arms, shoulders and hands afterward. As your strength and endurance improve, you can add variety, intensity and duration to your workout.

KEEP YOUR HANDS HEALTHY

Between workouts, whether you're flexing your fingers on a tennis ball, a finger board or a live body, keep your hands clean, warm and dry. Wash them after each massage session and nourish them with a lotion or cream of your choice. I'm

▼ To further strengthen your fingers, consider investing in a finger board, designed to help mountain climbers strengthen their grips. Warm up your hands, wrists and forearms by hanging on the largest rounded holds. Proceed by moving slowly around the board, alternating from large to small holds.

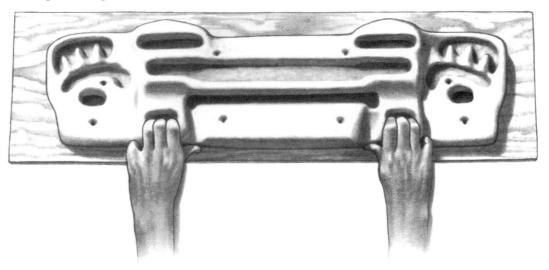

constantly trying new ones, though I have some favorites—Lubriderm, Nature's Gate and Biotone. Keep your nails trimmed and clean—I like to keep mine as short as possible, since I do a lot of deep-tissue work—and see a professional manicurist on occasion. If your hands are tired or particularly sore, ice them for 10 to 15 minutes and give them a day off from massage or working out.

Treat your hands to a hydrotherapy treatment from time to time, too: Soak in a bathtub or hot tub, or just let your hands dangle in warm water. Water is great therapy for your hands—or your whole body, for that matter. If I've had a particularly long day and have given many massages, I like to take a long, relaxing bath.

Even with the best of care, professional therapists sometimes develop arthritis in the fingers or wrists, and chronic problems can degenerate into carpal tunnel syndrome. This occurs when the nerves in the wrist become impinged or twisted, which leads to tingling in the hands and fingers. You can help avoid these ailments by using your body weight to augment the power of your hands. Learn to lean your whole body weight gently into the massage, and you will keep fresh hands and a healthy back and achieve a more flowing style. If you experience any significant discomfort during or after a session, such as pain in your neck, arms or hands, however, you should consult a doctor, a physical therapist or both.

As important as developing your hands is learning how to interpret what these most subtle of tools tell you. Massage is a two-way communication, with both giver and receiver focusing their awareness on the physical contact. People new to giving massages may be nervous at first, and they can transmit this discomfort to the person being massaged. If you become nervous while giving a massage, don't worry—after you've done a few massages you'll relax. Learning how to touch people in a healthy way is one of the great parts about caring in our lives. Starting with a friend makes giving a massage that much easier.

THE ULTIMATE TOOL

Think of your hands as extensions of your eyes and ears: Allow your hands to question your friend's body and listen to what they tell you. Explore the texture and depth of the muscles. Are they tight or loose? Thick or thin? Formless or distinct? Smooth or rough? Healthy or injured? Expand on what your hands learn by questioning your friend. Ask "Is this pressure right?" and "Is anything in particular bothering you?" Let your hands do most of the talking, but check things out verbally as well, especially when you're working on someone you've never massaged before.

I discuss specific techniques in chapter 4, but here are a few tips central to the art of massage.

Warm your hands. You can use running warm or hot water, or a moist, hot towel. You can also warm your lotion or oil by placing it in a tub of hot water. Always apply the oil, lotion or cream to your hands first. Then spread it on the person you're massaging, using a long, smooth stroke. You might also rub your hands together to warm them before beginning. And don't forget to remove your watch and rings—nothing chills a warm touch like a hunk of cold metal.

Relax your body and mind. Keep your hands loose, supple and flexible as they move. Think of yourself as a potter working clay; I like to think of myself as working on a living sculpture. Keep your hands in contact with the body as you move from one part to another; envision your hands as a mountain stream shaping itself to fit the rocks and boulders in its path. Let go of your own thoughts and keep your mind focused on the session.

Keep the pressure comfortable. All massage should begin with light to moderate pressure. As you gradually increase the depth of the strokes, watch your friend carefully to be sure that the pressure is not uncomfortable. Some of my clients describe successfully walking this fine line as "hurting good." Never assume that body size or gender defines just where this line is—everyone is different.

Vary the pressure. Ask your friend how the pressure feels and make sure that you spend some time getting massaged yourself to keep yourself aware of this important component. Gradually make changes in the movements of your body and your hands. Don't stop and start; just flow, staying smooth and relaxed. Explore different speeds and pressures as you learn new techniques and styles. Rhythm is an important component, and changing your style and technique regularly will help keep you from having problems with soreness or repetitive motion syndromes, which can occur when you do the same motion over and over again.

Shift your position as needed. I like working with my clients on a table, both because I find it more comfortable to shift my weight from one foot to the other and because I can get more leverage. Try standing with your feet shoulder-width apart and your knees slightly bent. If you're doing a massage on the floor, use padding under yourself and your friend. Giving a massage while sitting and kneeling requires practice: You can't get the power you can get while leaning your body weight into the strokes when standing, and it's more difficult to move around. Also, your body simply gets more tired by kneeling and squatting than by standing. But by keeping aware of your own comfort, whether standing or on the floor, you will learn to move with more precision and economy of effort.

Be spontaneous. Let your fingers do the thinking. I discovered some of my favorite techniques this way. Making up your own strokes is only a matter of imagination. There is no one official way to do massage. When you allow yourself freedom in discovering or creating new strokes, you will find yourself becoming more innovative.

You'll find the classical rendition of basic strokes in chapter 4, but you can combine these with two or more strokes to develop your own style. That's how massage, with all its diversity and various techniques, developed in the first place.

Pay attention to what you feel. Here's an exercise that can help your hands develop a feel for massage. I still use it frequently. Place your hands on one of your legs and use long, gliding strokes down the leg, focusing on the heels of your hands, then the palms, then the fingers and thumbs. Now gently stroke the other leg. Do you notice a difference between them? The leg you massaged thoroughly should feel relaxed and supple to the touch, and if you stretch out, you'll also find that the massaged leg is more flexible.

Now add variety, mixing techniques and pressures, while focusing on how these styles feel. Once you become fluent in the language of your hands, you'll be better able to communicate your knowledge to others.

CHAPTER

3

TOOLS OF THE TRADE

Every tool carries with it the spirit by which it has been created.

WERNER KARL HEISENBERG, *Physics and Philosophy*

A pair of caring and sensitive hands is all you need to begin practicing massage. But almost as important is the atmosphere you create and the environment you choose.

One of the goals of sports massage is to create a level of comfort for reduced muscle tension and a deep level of physical and psychological relaxation—the more comfortable the setting, the more effective the massage. Before giving a massage, you'll want to carefully assess the physical surroundings. Is the room warm enough? Do you and the person you're going to massage feel comfortable? Do you have everything you need so you won't have to interrupt the flow of the session?

Let's look at the necessary ingredients for a satisfying massage. I'll start with the setting, consider the work surface, then discuss lubricants and tools.

CHOOSE THE SCENE

The more comfortable the setting, the more effective the massage. The two essential ingredients are warmth and quiet. Choose a room that is airy and peaceful. If you have a spare room, you could set this up for massage so it's available anytime. And I never rule out doing massage outdoors, if weather permits—near the ocean, by a river or mountain stream or simply under a tree in the backyard. Arrange freshly washed blankets, sheets and towels and any oils and tools you plan to use close by; I like to keep a tote bag full of necessary items ready to go. Keep cushions or pillows within reach. You can kneel or sit on them or place them under your friend's body to ease tense spots. Remember, comfort is as important to the receiver as it is to the giver. You need to be comfortable so the person you are massaging will receive your uninterrupted attention.

Soft lighting is ideal; lighted candles or a crackling fire lends emotional as well as physical warmth. You can use those blankets, sheets and towels if your friend becomes chilly or as a cover when the massage is complete. Warmth is vital to your friend's comfort! Remember that when we're lying down relaxed, our heart rates and body temperatures fall—and lubricants used in massage may make the skin feel cooler. So preheat the room if necessary, then maintain a temperature between 70° and 74°F.

SELECTING A WORK SURFACE

For proper massage, you need a firm surface. A bed won't do—your friend will sink in the marshmallow softness of the mattress! You can choose a table specifically built for this purpose—which I recommend if you intend to do massage regularly—or you can use the floor.

It's possible to give a great massage on a pad on the floor, and it won't be tiring for you or uncomfortable for your friend if you go about it the right way. But on the floor you'll have to tailor techniques a bit: You can't move around as freely, and you'll probably want to cut the session short to spare yourself stiffness. Listen to your back and knees!

If the floor is well-carpeted, you will need only an egg crate–style foam pad, which you can find at any department store, and a clean sheet to cover the floor. If the floor isn't carpeted, you'll want a foam pad at least three inches thick. You could use a couple of sleeping bags or a futon as a substitute for the pad. In any case, make sure the padding extends well beyond your friend on the sides and ends so that your knees will be protected, and you won't end up needing a massage yourself! A 7-by-4-foot surface should be adequate.

A table is the best choice, however, and it's wise to invest in one especially made for massage. While you could modify an old kitchen table, massage tables are specifically designed with both giver and receiver in mind. They're built so that you can adjust them to the right height to allow you maximum leverage while massaging, so you're less likely to strain your back. If the table is equipped with a face cradle—which I highly recommend—you'll have easier access to the head, neck, shoulders and back while massaging someone who is facedown. The back, shoulders, neck and head will be well-supported, so most techniques that are tricky to do comfortably on the floor can be performed with ease. And on a table, you can perform additional techniques that require more room, such as certain range-of-motion stretches you'll find detailed in chapter 4.

You can choose either a permanent table or a portable one that will allow

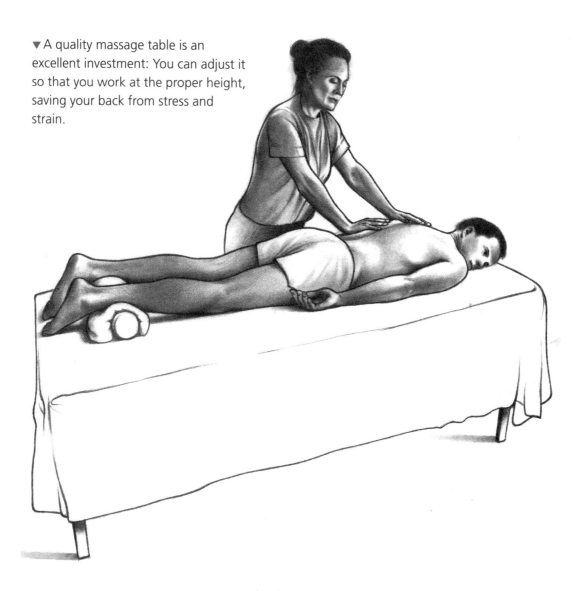

▼ A quality massage table is an excellent investment: You can adjust it so that you work at the proper height, saving your back from stress and strain.

. . . .

THE BUILD-IT-YOURSELF OPTION

Unless you're an experienced woodworker, you'll likely find making your own massage table a formidable challenge, and you may find your creation less comfortable, stable and inexpensive than you'd hoped. If you want to save a few bucks, and you favor a quick and easy approach to construction, however, here are two alternatives.

- Make or buy two sawhorses 28 to 32 inches high and 28 inches wide. Buy a piece of ¾-inch plywood, have it cut to 28 inches by 73 inches and cut a 3-inch-thick foam pad to the same length. Nail and glue the plywood to the top of the sawhorses. Then place the foam pad on top, covered with a clean sheet.

- Order a massage table kit. Stronglite has an excellent one for around $200. Contact Stronglite Massage Table Kits, 255 Davidson Street, Cottage Grove, OR 97424; 1-800-289-5487.

. . . .

you to do massage anywhere. Standard tables measure 29 to 32 inches wide and 73 inches long and weigh 20 to 30 pounds. When you buy a table, select one that best meets your needs, such as the amount of space you have available and whether you want to carry your table to other settings. I suggest that you don't try to cut corners: Used tables from the 1960s, 1970s and 1980s may seem like a bargain, but they're typically heavy and may creak and shake. It's better to choose one of the newer models: These tables, typically made of pine, oak or maple, collapse handily for easy storage and portability and can easily be set up by one person. Costs can range from as little as $200 to $800 or more, depending on the model and its options.

Where do you find tables? Occasionally, you can find a good used table in classified ads or through a local massage school. Before buying a used table, check out how easy it is to set up and move around and how well it supports a person's weight. For new ones, look for advertisements in health magazines. I support companies with an environmental commitment and hope you will, too. There's no need to harm the planet while we heal ourselves! Look for table makers that use chlorofluorocarbon-free upholstery foam, northern hardwoods and water-based lacquers.

Here are several companies that sell massage tables in their catalogs.

• The Massage Store, Ltd., also known as Colorado Healing Arts Products, P.O. Box 2247, Boulder, CO 80306; 1-800-728-2426

• Golden Ratio Woodworks, P.O. Box 297, Emigrant, MT 59027; 1-800-345-1129

• Living Earths Crafts, 600 East Todd Road, Santa Rosa, CA 95407; 1-800-358-8292

• Oakworks, Inc., P.O. Box 99, Glen Rock, PA 17327-0099; 1-800-558-8850

SETTING THE RIGHT HEIGHT

The height of the massage table is important; state-of-the-art tables adjust from 20 to 44 inches. Set your table too low, and you can strain your back; set it too high, and you won't have the leverage you need. Over the years, I've gradually lowered my table—not because I'm shrinking with age, but because I've experimented with height and leverage and found that for me a lower height just works better.

To adjust your table correctly, stand straight with your shoulders level. Extend both arms down with your hands at right angles to your forearms. Your palms should be level with the table surface, which should be about at the top of your thighs. As you do more and more massages, you can tinker with the table height to find the height that feels best for you.

GETTING INTO POSITION

Take care not to neglect your own body while caring for someone else's: It's crucial to use good posture and the right equipment, ease your own tensions and breathe smoothly and fully. Your spine should feel lengthened—do not overstretch or round your shoulders. A balanced body awareness will give your movements grace and power and help you finish a session feeling refreshed.

Breathing fully will help you relax and release any lingering mental and emotional stress. Encourage this in the person you're massaging, too. Slow, deep and steady breaths help you focus on the session, supply oxygen to the body and calm your mind.

CHOOSING YOUR LUBRICANT

There will be times when you won't want to use a lubricant, such as during shiatsu massage (see page 28) or clothed sessions and before or after workouts or races. (Oils interfere with the skin's cooling mechanisms and may feel greasy.) Most techniques used in nude or draped sessions require some lubricant, however, and you may find the array of choices available to you overwhelming at first.

For beginners, I'd suggest using an inexpensive and easy-to-find oil. Many inexpensive lubricants are available. Cold-pressed vegetable oils make a good choice for full-body massage and have the benefit of bringing natural nutrients to the skin. They include walnut, peanut, coconut and safflower oils and can be found at most grocery stores or natural food stores. You can add a few teaspoons of more luxurious oils, such as peach or avocado, to enrich the mix; a teaspoon of wheat-germ oil in your base will keep it from turning rancid. You can find peach, avocado and wheat-germ oils at body-and-bath stores.

Some oils, such as mineral and baby oils, either clog the pores or are absorbed too easily by the skin and need to be reapplied frequently to maintain a slick surface. The same is true with most hand lotions. This isn't optimal, because numerous applications will interrupt the session, disrupting both your rhythm and the mood.

As you explore different lubricants, you'll find that viscosity and workability vary widely. Coconut oil is heavy, for example, while almond oil is lighter. What choice will make the going smooth for you and the person you're massaging? It's a matter of personal preference. Does it feel good on the skin? If it's scented, is the smell appealing? Does it require repeated applications? Is it suited for recovery or for deep-tissue work? Bear in mind that preferences vary, and a scent you enjoy may annoy the person you're massaging. Also, some people are sensitive to certain fragrances, so you should always ask before the first session.

There is no perfect lubricant. My preferences have evolved over the years, and I'll always try something new. I prefer the gliding feel you can get from creams; to me, oils feel too thin. Creams and salves are preferable for deep-tissue work because they allow more friction.

My all-time favorite product for all purposes is Dual-Purpose Massage Creme by Biotone. To me, it provides the optimum balance between the workability of an oil and the absorption of a lotion: It has more glide than a lotion, and it leaves a soft, smooth feel without any residue on the skin. One of its ingredients is the wildflower arnica, which helps skin circulation and is restorative to sore muscles. At this writing, a 14-ounce container sells for around $15 and will last for two dozen massages.

Store your oils and lotions in spill-proof plastic bottles with either a lock-top lid or a pump. You can buy bottles at drugstores, cosmetic stores, natural food stores or five-and-dimes. Better yet, recycle one from home. You can keep creams and salves in any large, lidded container. You can store spare lubricants fresh in the refrigerator, but you must warm them to room temperature before you use them! Set them out one hour before the massage, or warm them by immersing the bottle in a bowl of

• •

USING SCENTS AND HERBS

Some people like to use various herbs or plant extracts during massage, either mixed in with salves or combined with oils, either for a therapeutic effect or simply because they like the aroma.

You may want to experiment with herbal lubricants. Comfrey, sage, calendula and arnica can be used in oils, salves or creams. You can buy these in the form of oils or salves and then add them to your base lubricant. I customarily use these herbs—particularly arnica—to help people recover from soreness.

In aromatherapy, the essences of certain plants are extracted as essential oils and then applied to the skin, burned as incense or taken by mouth. These essences can be refreshing and invigorating or soothing and relaxing, and applied externally, may help reduce muscular aches and fatigue. Like massage, aromatherapy has a long history, but scientists are just beginning to study the correlation between scent and wellness.

Essences commonly used in sports massage for treating muscular fatigue include eucalyptus, peppermint, wintergreen, birch and ginger. Aromatherapists believe that lavender, mandarin and roman chamomile have calming qualities and that clove, cinnamon and thyme have anti-inflammatory effects.

Personally, I prefer to use an unscented cream for massage because my skin tends to be allergic to many substances. Instead of applying the scent directly, I may use a vaporizer and add just enough oil to gently scent the room.

Explore and experiment; create your own mixes. A word of caution: Always ask about allergies or sensitivities before trying a scent or herb; keep in mind that children and the elderly tend to have sensitive skin. And since essential oils can be absorbed into the skin, and certain herbs have strong medicinal effects, it's a good idea for women who are pregnant or breastfeeding or people with epilepsy, high blood pressure, cancer, HIV or AIDS, asthma, allergies or sensitive skin to check with their physicians before undergoing massage with essential oils.

• •

warm water. Spare your friend from being chilled out of his senses when he had expected a warm, nurturing massage.

You can find oils, lotions, salves and cream lubricants at specialty stores, or you can order them from one of these companies.

- Biotone, 4564 Alvarado Canyon Road #1, San Diego, CA 92120; 1-800-445-6457

- Everybody, Ltd., 1175 Walnut Street, Boulder, CO 80302; 1-800-748-5675

- The Massage Store, Ltd., P.O. Box 2247, Boulder, CO 80306; 1-800-728-2426

You should thoroughly wash your hands before and after any session; whatever soap you like to use is fine. After a session, take care not to rub your eyes or handle food or drink before washing your hands. And your friend may want to shower off the lubricant afterward. Some lubricants tend to stain or soil linen and clothing—although the effects of the products I have mentioned are minimal—so showering is a good idea.

SETTING THE MOOD WITH MUSIC

With the area ready and your lubricant selected, you can add a final touch with music, if you like. Research shows that music can help us relax more quickly. The key is choosing the right selection—not every piece works for everyone. Piano, flute and harp are good bets, however, and recordings of nature sounds also work. Experiment, and if the music feels good to you and your friend, keep listening.

One of the best massages I ever received was accompanied by Tibetan flute music. At the end of the relaxing hour-and-a-half session, I imagined I was in Tibet at 10,000 feet. Actually, I was a mere 6,000 feet above sea level in a Boulder massage office. Such is the power of music in tandem with touch.

Here are some of my favorite selections. (Look for them at your favorite music store or order through a massage catalog.)

- *Music to Disappear In*, Rafael. Piano, synthesizer, flute, guitar, percussion; side one is uplifting, angelic and orchestral, while side two is tribal and trancelike.

- *Spectrum Suite*, Steven Halpern. Electric piano; the "antifrantic" alternative—soothing and healing music.

- *Conferring with the Moon*, William Ackerman. Acoustic guitar, strings, piano, woodwinds, synthesizer; light and relaxing, with weaving and repeating melodies.

- *Land of Enchantment*, Deuter. Native flute, acoustic guitar, synthesizer, sounds of nature.

- *Aboriginal Sound and Feel of South American Indian Flutes*. An inspirational piece.

- *Manatee Dreams of Neptune*, Emerald Web. A smooth blend of synthesizers, percussion and flutes that exudes warmth and elegance.

- *Pianoscapes*, Michael Jones. "Landscape portraits" through piano; contemporary music that creates images of rolling hills and open fields.

- *Woodlands*, Narada. Piano and guitar pieces.

- *Between Tides*, Roger Eno. Distinctive piano music accompanied by strings, flute and clarinet.

If you prefer more rhythm, try one of these.

- *Nouveau Flamenco*, Ottmar Liebert. Guitar; a spirited and uplifting selection.

- *Bhakti Point*, Richard Burmer. Exotic sounds mixed with proportioned melodies.

- *Traveler*, Paul Horn. Flute and rhythm; varying tempos throughout.

- *Inside the Taj Mahal*, Paul Horn. More great flute pieces, recorded at the Taj Mahal.

- *Tibet*, Mark Isham. Rhythmic forms of haiku.

- *Autumn*, George Winston. Rhythmic, strong piano compositions with a whole range of tempos throughout. Any of Winston's work is a sure bet.

- *Rainforest*, Jerry Garcia. Gentle piano and guitar with synthesized strings; slow to medium tempos.

- *Deep Breakfast*, Ray Lynch. Electrical and acoustic instrumentation; light, bouncy and playful.

- *Cicada*, Deuter. Native flute, acoustic guitar, synthesizer, bells and natural sounds.

TAKING THE NEXT STEP

Once you've established a massage routine, you may want to add some massage tools to your routine. You can use body tools as an extension of massaging with your hands, on yourself as well as on another person. Tools effectively help reduce muscle tension and will become a welcome part of your self-care program and massage style. The beauty of these devices is that people love to use them. People are more likely to follow through with a self-care program when it feels great. And who doesn't like massage?

I have found many of the following tools to be effective, economical, environmentally conscious and sturdy. Prices noted may change after publication.

- The Thera Cane is my all-time favorite. It is a deep-pressure device that gently massages tender points in the muscles that often develop from poor posture, stress or overwork. Each Thera Cane comes with an illustrated manual to show you how to massage the back, neck, shoulders, arms and legs. With the Thera Cane, there is no place on your back that you can't reach! It weighs one pound and is made of fiberglass. Cost: around $30. (For more about the Thera Cane, see chapter 5.)

- The Knobble is a rounded wooden device that saves wear and tear on your hands and thumbs while addressing trigger points through deep-pressure techniques. Cost: around $10.

- The Thumbsaver is a small wooden ball with a projecting rubber knob that you use to apply direct pressure-point massage to the face, neck, shoulders, arms and legs. It's easy to use and portable. Cost: around $5.

- The Foot Massage is one of the finest tools I've used. It was designed by a reflexologist—a specialist who targets "zones" in the feet that correspond to specific body parts. It's a 9-by-2-inch wooden dowel with raised, hard plastic bumps. Cost: around $20.

- The Thera Stick is a long wooden tool with two plastic "balls" attached that firmly press and stretch the spine's supporting muscles to relieve tension all the way up and down your back. Cost: around $20.

- The Acu-Reflex Massager is a "pain eraser" made of natural rubber with 38 acupressure "fingers" on two knobby balls attached to a plastic handle. It stimulates circulation and relieves stress all over the body. Cost: around $20.

- Bioscape Mattress Pads are the finest quality egg crate–style foam available. Use these to give a comfortable massage on the floor; just cover with a sheet. Cost: around $50.

You can look for these tools in specialty stores or look for ads in health or massage magazines. Here are a few sources that carry many massage and massage-related products.

- The Massage Store, Ltd., P.O. Box 2247, Boulder, CO 80306; 1-800-728-2426

- SelfCare Catalog, P.O. Box 8813, Emeryville, CA 94608; 1-800-345-3371

- Stretching Inc., P.O. Box 767, Palmer Lake, CO 80133; 1-800-333-1307

Many other tools are available, and new ones will always be created. You'll find those that are mentioned here to be among the most rewarding—and they'll be your friends for years to come. So knead your neck, cushion your feet, roll away muscle tension and remember the proverb from Benjamin Franklin: "God heals, and the doctor takes the fee."

Now you know about the generous range of massage tools. As you begin practicing, you'll become more confident about where, when and how to apply them. When you're first becoming acquainted with this healing art, it's natural to concentrate on getting everything exactly right. As you become more comfortable with all your tools and techniques, you can start massaging in a less regimented and more instinctual way.

Once we give ourselves permission to trust our hands, touch becomes a natural healing and empathy between human beings. Trust your feelings and responses. You'll find yourself giving flowing, caring massages that acknowledge your wholeness as well as that of the friend beneath your hands.

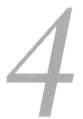

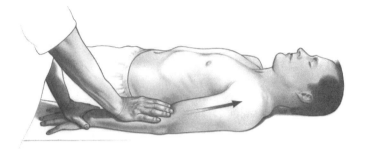

C H A P T E R

MASSAGE TECHNIQUES MADE EASY

Athletes—the ones who last for very long, anyway—eventually
come to understand that the single physical asset most critical to
continued and successful hard use of the human body isn't strength
or speed or endurance, but suppleness.

JOHN JEROME, *Staying Supple*

Massage techniques, like stretching techniques, are relatively easy to grasp. Let's start with four common techniques: effleurage, friction, petrissage and tapotement.

Effleurage. This technique is used to stretch and relax the muscles, get tissue fluids moving and create intramuscular motion to stretch adhesions, the fibrous materials, usually resulting from injury, that bind one muscle fiber to another and restrict the natural range of motion. Effleurage uses the fingers and the flat of the hand in long, gliding strokes directed toward the heart (see page 26). This motion helps the circulation of venous blood and lymph fluid, a bloodlike substance that removes bacteria and transports fat from the intestines.

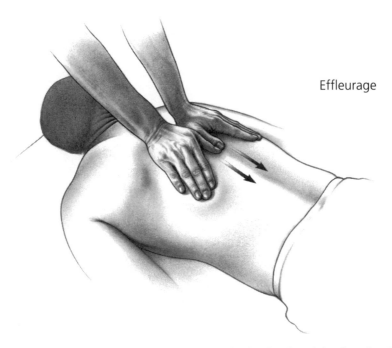

Effleurage

Friction. Friction involves bracing with the heels of the hands, then moving the fingers or thumbs in a circle. It's used around joints and on tough areas such as scars, knots or muscle spasms. In cross-fiber massage, also called deep transverse friction, you use your thumb or fingertips to apply pressure slowly across an area of a muscle or tendon at roughly a 90-degree angle as shown below, moving the fingers with the skin, not over it. The thicker the muscle or tendon, the harder you push.

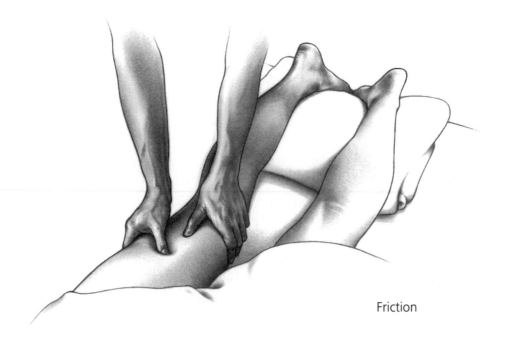

Friction

Petrissage. Like effleurage, petrissage relaxes and stretches muscles, helps move tissue fluids and stretches adhesions. It requires a grabbing stroke similar to the motion used to knead bread. You squeeze, compress and roll the tissues; it's used primarily on areas such as the trapezius, the latissimus dorsi or the triceps (see pages 30 and 31 to identify muscle groups). Compression is a variant of petrissage, using the palm of one hand with the other hand on top for leverage, pushing directly down into the belly, or fullest part, of the muscle.

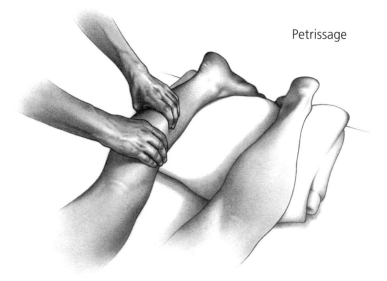

Petrissage

Tapotement. This is a striking stroke performed by either cupping (below) or hacking (page 28). Cupping uses a light tapping or slapping motion with the palms of the hands cupped, which stimulates the area to increase circulation. This can be followed by hacking with the edges of your hands.

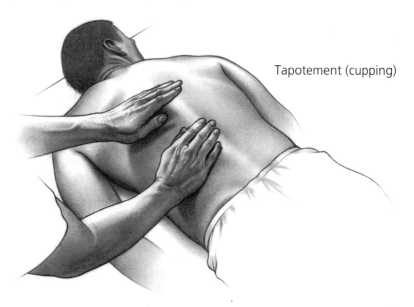

Tapotement (cupping)

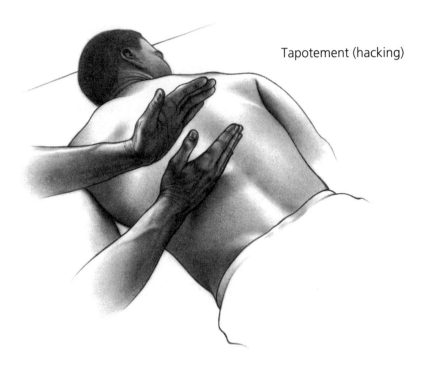

Tapotement (hacking)

BASIC MASSAGE STYLES

All styles of massage—Swedish, deep-tissue, trigger-point and shiatsu—use one or more of these techniques.

- Swedish massage combines effleurage, kneading and friction on the surface of the muscles with assisted movement of the joints. It relaxes the mind and body, warms up and flushes toxins out of the muscles and improves circulation and range of motion.

- Deep-tissue massage, as its name implies, uses slow strokes and deep hand pressure on tight areas, either following or going against the grain of the muscles, tendons and fascia (the connective tissues that cover, support and connect the muscles and the inner organs). It releases patterns of tension and restores suppleness and length.

- Trigger-point therapy applies concentrated finger pressure on "trigger points" to break the cycle of spasm and pain. Trigger points are small, very sensitive areas in the muscle fibers that develop under extreme physical stress, commonly in the lower back, neck and shoulders. You locate trigger points with gentle probing.

- Shiatsu is massage blended with acupressure. Pressure is applied to special points along meridians, the invisible channels of energy flow in the body; you can think of it as acupuncture without needles.

Two other disciplines that go beyond the scope of this book deserve brief mention. Reflexology uses principles similar to those of shiatsu but is organized around a system of certain points on the hands and feet that correspond to other areas of the body. Rolfing, named after its developer, Ida Rolf, is deep muscular manipulation and massage that can be painful (see page 148). It's intended to relieve physical and emotional tension and align the body structurally. It can often restore muscle length and suppleness even in chronic cases.

You may prefer one style, or incorporate several for a more eclectic "feel." Regardless of your preferred style, remember that sports massage doesn't require much movement or many strokes. It's more important to create a deep, gentle pressure. Also, it's best to stroke toward the heart whenever possible to aid lymph and venous blood flow.

LET THE BODY BE YOUR GUIDE

The signals and sensations we get from the body as it's being massaged are valuable messages. The pain is telling you something. So is the pleasure. Breathe deeply as you learn to relax completely. And remember—a good massage is one given with a sense of direction and purpose actually felt by the recipient.

When you're considering which technique or combination of techniques to use, consider not only your friend's response to what you're doing, but also his or her condition and needs. Sports massage targets specific muscle groups, and the amount of time spent working on a given group depends on how much and when the athlete uses it. Extended deep-tissue work such as friction petrissage could hurt an athlete's performance if given just before a competition. Similarly, a brief tapotement session, because it involves such a light touch, would be inadequate to flush out toxins and relax muscles after a grueling effort.

I experienced this in my professional practice: Cross-country runner Gwyn Coogan was training to qualify for the January 1993 World Championships when she became my client. Noting a number of little overuse injuries, including shin-splints, plantar fasciitis and mild tendinitis, that threatened to sideline Gwyn, I spoke with Mark Plaatjes, who's a physical therapist as well as a world-class marathoner. Between us we developed a preventive approach that included deep-tissue work, physical therapy, hydrotherapy and a change in shoes and orthotics.

At first, I did relatively little deep-tissue work on Gwyn—just enough to begin to normalize the tissues—because I didn't want to interfere with her performance at the U.S. Championships, which came before the Worlds. Deep-tissue work effectively restructures your muscles and can initially make you feel sluggish.

After she made the national team, and with six weeks before the Worlds, I was able to work more aggressively to eliminate remaining muscular problems and build Gwyn's resistance to those small but numerous injuries. As the race neared, the deep-tissue work no longer left her lethargic. Ultimately, Gwyn was able to compete healthy and injury-free at the Worlds. Her performance wasn't all she had hoped for, but she wasn't sidelined by her injuries. It turned out that she was three months pregnant at the time.

Take your time; begin gently and give the muscles a chance to relax. As the

MUSCLE GROUPS: FRONT VIEW

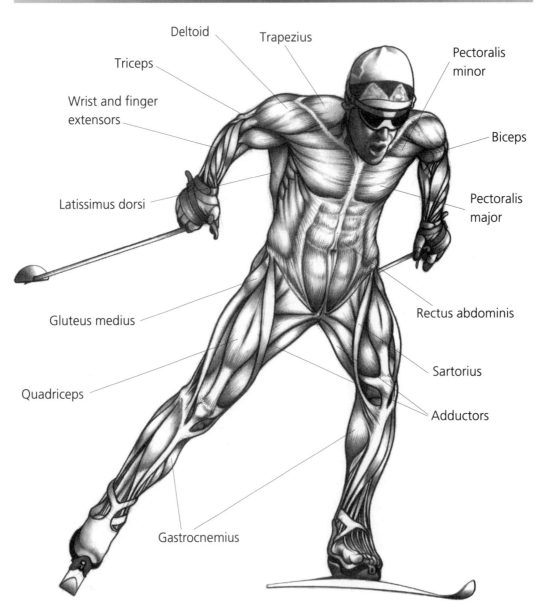

Deltoid
Trapezius
Pectoralis minor
Triceps
Wrist and finger extensors
Biceps
Latissimus dorsi
Pectoralis major
Rectus abdominis
Gluteus medius
Sartorius
Quadriceps
Adductors
Gastrocnemius

tissues begin to adjust and let go, the massage will become more pleasurable for the recipient. At that point you can gradually increase the pressure. Use a slow, deep, kneading movement; as tension and soreness seem to shift, you can gradually release the pressure and move on to another spot. Whether you're giving or receiving the massage, remember to focus on and breathe deeply into those tense spots; your goal should be to relax completely.

MUSCLE GROUPS: BACK VIEW

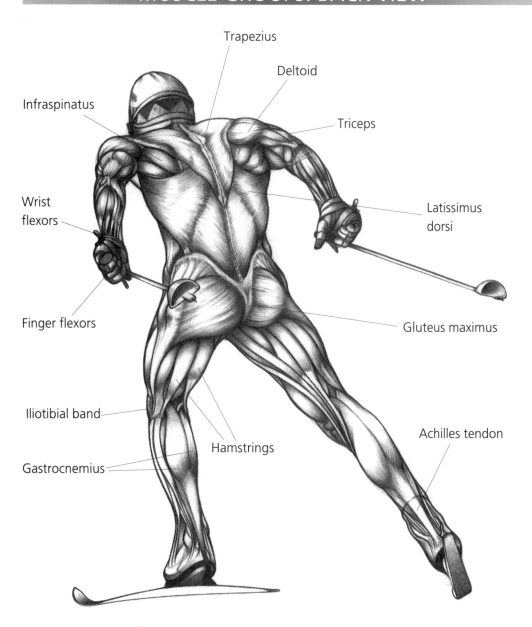

Trapezius

Deltoid

Infraspinatus

Triceps

Wrist flexors

Latissimus dorsi

Finger flexors

Gluteus maximus

Iliotibial band

Hamstrings

Gastrocnemius

Achilles tendon

A MATTER OF TIMING

If you begin to closely observe the body—noting pleasure, pain and the other signals that it sends—you'll gradually learn when a particular technique is called for and when one should be avoided. There's no shortcut to learning this, but a general rule is to stay away from new or more vigorous techniques directly before competition.

You'll also come to recognize signs of overtraining—in yourself and in friends—and learn how to combine massage and cross-training techniques to stay fit while keeping injuries to a minimum. Athletes such as Gwyn learn from experience. She is finding the right balance between training and racing, family life and studying for a Ph.D. in higher mathematics—while making time for preventive care.

You'll also come to appreciate how the timing of a massage affects performance. Here are some general suggestions for massages both before and after activity.

Pre-event massage. Don't use any oil for massages immediately before activity, because oil can interfere with the skin's cooling mechanisms, and the oily sensation may be unpleasant during activity. Use light, brisk, vigorous strokes to soften and warm the muscles, increase circulation and maintain suppleness. Use a blend of petrissage, compression and tapotement. Work for 15 to 30 minutes.

Concentrate on areas of the body of particular concern. A cyclist might want to focus the pre-event massage on preparing the quadriceps for intense activity; a skier suffering from pre-race tension might favor the neck and shoulders. Consider what works best for that particular athlete before an event—this may include warm-up, stretching and mind/body connection routines.

Post-event massage. Oil is optional for massages done within 12 hours of activity. Use long, gliding strokes. Avoid deep strokes, which can cause muscle tears or add to damage already done by hard efforts.

Experts believe that the increased circulation created by a post-event massage helps flush out toxins that cause soreness and stiffness. This reduces the time needed for recovery from intense exertion, cutting recovery by as much as one-half; some of the athletes I massage report recovery in 24 hours rather than 48 hours. Work for 30 to 60 minutes. As in pre-race massage, give special attention to problem areas.

Curative/restorative massage. Oils or salves are normally used in this full-body, deep-tissue massage, which is done 24 to 72 hours after activity and uses the entire repertoire of strokes. The curative/restorative massage keeps muscles stretched and restores elasticity and suppleness. It also prevents toxin buildup and softens fibrous tissue. Work for one to two hours, concentrating on problem areas.

If an event was particularly strenuous—say, a marathon—you may want to do a Swedish-style massage on yourself or on your friend and delay a deep-tissue massage until the following week. This will give you or your friend time to recover from soreness.

WHEN *NOT* TO GIVE (OR GET) A MASSAGE

Contrary to what you might assume it's not wise to massage someone who feels physically ill or is in severe pain—doing so could aggravate an injury or illness. Likewise, you don't want to massage someone immediately after an injury has occurred, while tissues are severely damaged.

Also do not massage:

• Acute inflammation or bruising
• Any area where there is new scar tissue or undiagnosed lumps or swellings
• Directly over varicose veins
• Rashes, boils or open wounds

Check with a physician before massaging anyone who has:

• Cardiovascular or circulatory conditions, such as thrombosis or phlebitis, or any type of coronary disease
• Diabetes, particularly in advanced stages
• Acute back pain, severe injury, fever or high blood pressure
• Conditions such as epilepsy, cancer, HIV or AIDS, or undiagnosed illness or disease

Massage during pregnancy is not advisable and should be done only if okayed by the physician of the mother-to-be. You should not massage a pregnant woman, however, if she is suffering nausea, vaginal bleeding, diarrhea or abdominal pain.

The same caveat applies if you're the one who isn't feeling well or has a health condition that rules out massage.

And by the way, if you have the flu, be sure to wait about a week after you've passed the contagious stage before getting a massage. Some people think that because their muscles ache when they have the flu, they'll feel better with a massage, but I've found that massage will actually make you feel *worse*. If, however, you only have a head cold , you may benefit from a massage, beginning with the face and moving toward the toes; this seems to help clear congestion.

Now that you know what to do and when, you're ready to start using some of these techniques and styles. Before you begin, it's a good idea to review chapters 2 and 3.

THE BACK

The best place to start learning massage is the back. The knowledge and experience gained there can easily be applied to the rest of the body. The whole back should take at least 20 minutes. Have the friend you're going to massage lie facedown. Cover the buttocks and legs with towels for warmth and comfort. (Many people prefer to remain covered or draped.) The illustrations in this book show common massage positions that give maximum comfort to both the giver and receiver.

If you're using oil, salve or cream, apply it to your palms to warm it and spread it over the back and shoulders and the sides of the torso. Less is better than too much—you can always apply additional oil or salve if it's needed.

▼ Standing at the head of the table or kneeling above your friend's head, place your palms at the top of the back with the edge of your palms on either side of the spine, but not on top of the spine itself. Let your hands glide down the entire length of the back to the top of the buttocks. This is an effleurage stroke. Use firm pressure, leaning into the strokes as you go. Reverse the hand position with the fingertips next to the spine. Repeat this six times. This is a classic stroke that you will frequently use to begin and end a session.

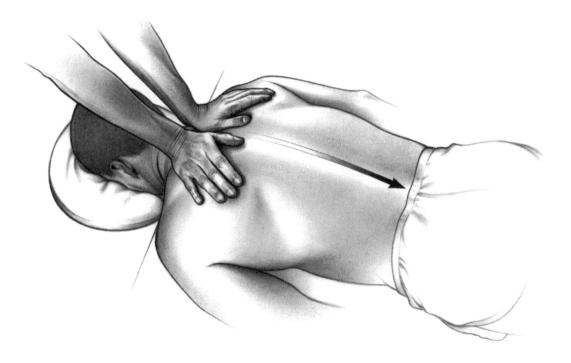

▼ Now, stand at the side of the table and use your elbow to work lightly along, but not on top of, the spine. Start at either the shoulders or buttocks; go slowly, carefully exploring pressure and speed. Repeat three times.

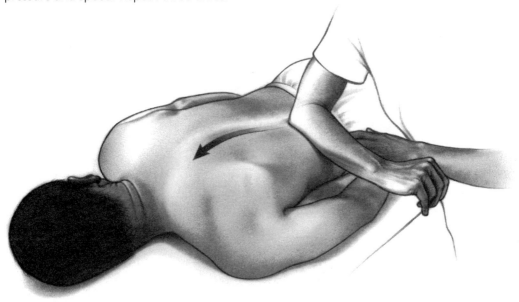

▼ You can now do some pulling along the sides of the torso. Reach across the table and work the side opposite you. Start at the buttocks and work your way up, with the fingers pointing down and the hands pulling up; find a comfortable rhythm. Work both sides in the same fashion.

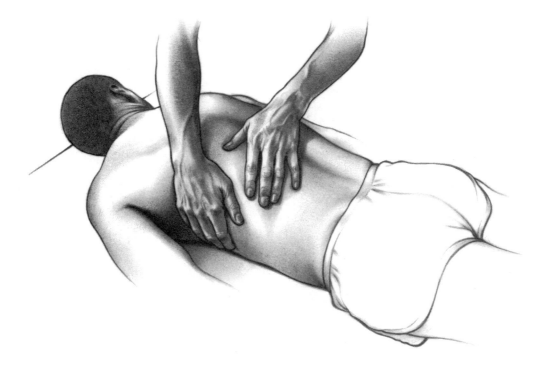

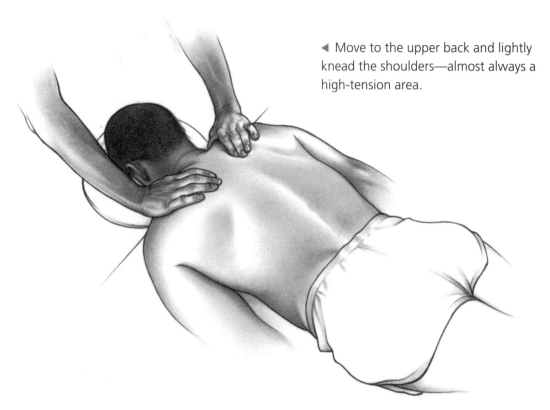

◄ Move to the upper back and lightly knead the shoulders—almost always a high-tension area.

▼ With the back now warmed up, you can proceed to medium-depth strokes and then on to deep-tissue strokes. At this point you will find the body less fragile than you might have thought. Remember, though, that people vary in what they find comfortable, so ask your friend for feedback. Starting at the top of the buttocks and using a friction stroke along the spine, make small, deep circles with your thumbs. Proceed to the base of the neck as shown until you reach the bottom ridge of the skull.

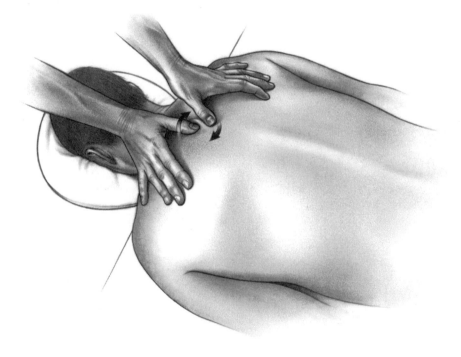

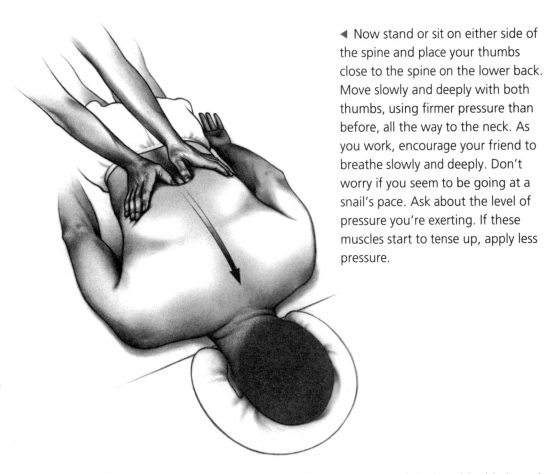

◄ Now stand or sit on either side of the spine and place your thumbs close to the spine on the lower back. Move slowly and deeply with both thumbs, using firmer pressure than before, all the way to the neck. As you work, encourage your friend to breathe slowly and deeply. Don't worry if you seem to be going at a snail's pace. Ask about the level of pressure you're exerting. If these muscles start to tense up, apply less pressure.

▼ Next, knead the sides of the back from the middle to the edge of the shoulder blade and again toward the lower back. Standing or sitting on the opposite side, reach across and grasp the side with both hands and knead in either direction. Repeat this three times on both sides.

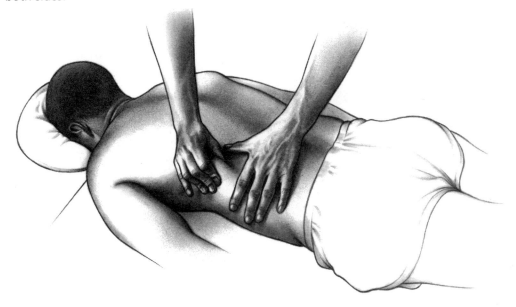

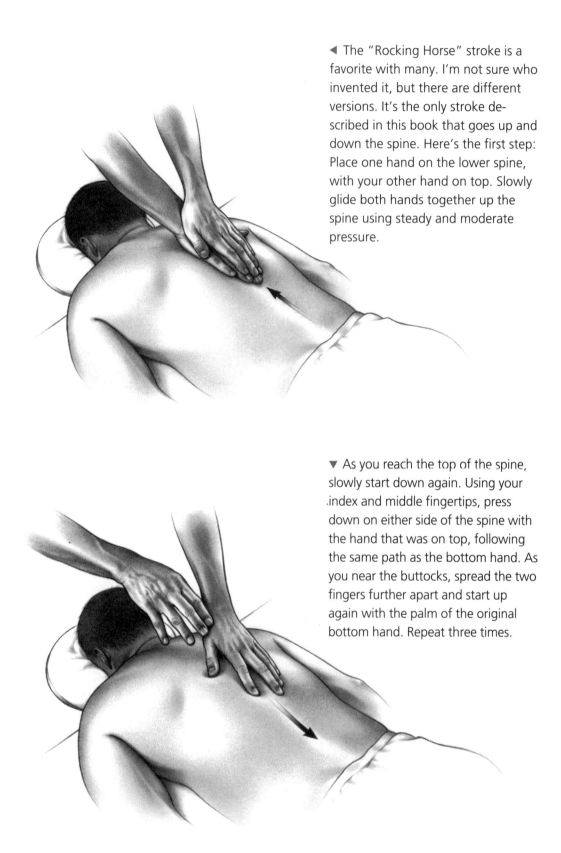

◀ The "Rocking Horse" stroke is a favorite with many. I'm not sure who invented it, but there are different versions. It's the only stroke described in this book that goes up and down the spine. Here's the first step: Place one hand on the lower spine, with your other hand on top. Slowly glide both hands together up the spine using steady and moderate pressure.

▼ As you reach the top of the spine, slowly start down again. Using your index and middle fingertips, press down on either side of the spine with the hand that was on top, following the same path as the bottom hand. As you near the buttocks, spread the two fingers further apart and start up again with the palm of the original bottom hand. Repeat three times.

▼ Next, work on the shoulder blades. First, ask to make sure that your friend has no history of shoulder separation or dislocation. Then, standing at either side of the table, gently place one of your friend's arms behind the back; this makes the shoulder blade very accessible. Lifting the blade, use your fingertips to pull it away from the underlying muscle group. (As I tell my brother, a professional chef, pretend you're filleting a chicken.) Pull up and away from the blade, working gently, and don't forget to ask your friend if the pressure is comfortable.

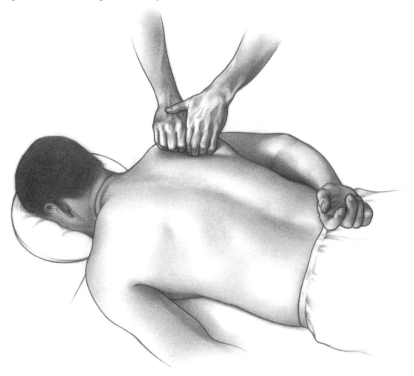

▼ Use the side of your hands as you would a knife; you can use your thumbs to probe tension spots. Repeat the process for the other shoulder blade.

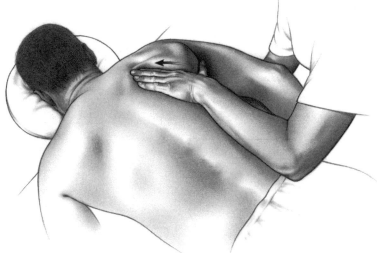

▼ Continue working on the shoulders, one at a time, from the base of the neck, kneading all the fleshy areas. Concentrate on little knots of tension you come across with your thumbs. Knead around the shoulder blade and the side of the rib cage; follow the contours. Continue to work on specific areas of tension that you find with your thumbs. Use small, firm strokes.

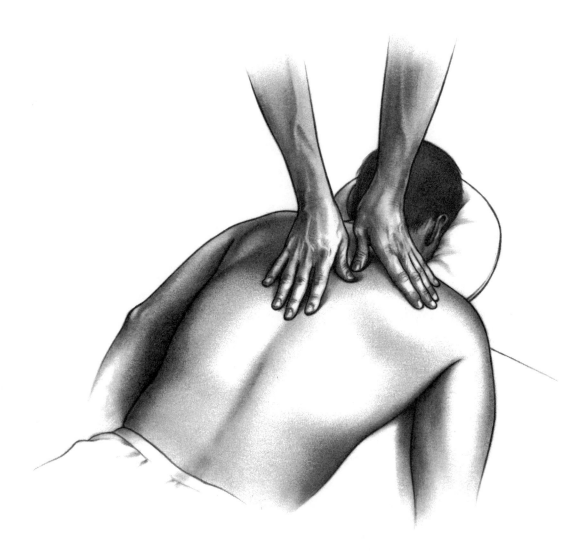

▼ Now work with your thumbs on the lower back. Use an alternating stroke on either side of the spine. Stay close to the spine, but not on top of it, with circular petrissage motions. Work the area (roughly the size of a softball). Repeat on the other side.

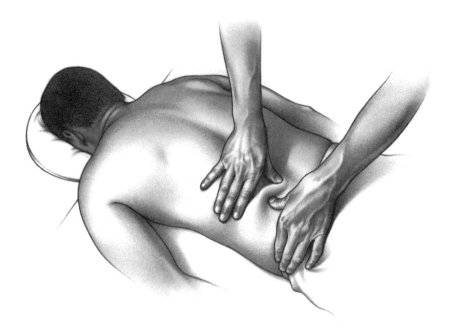

▼ Finally, place your forearms flat on the middle of the back. Begin with the forearms close together, then spread them away from each other, one moving toward the shoulders, the other toward the buttocks.

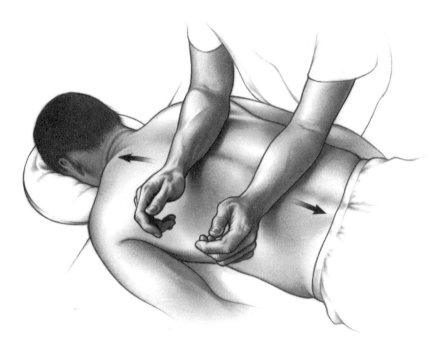

THE BUTTOCKS AND THE BACKS OF THE LEGS

As you exercise, the juncture of the buttocks and legs is the center of power and control, so it's important to work this area thoroughly. You will complete the massage on the back of the body by finishing with the legs and feet.

The legs are especially important to athletes who make heavy use of the lower body, such as runners, skiers, cyclists, hikers, skaters and triathletes. The back of the leg contains the hamstrings, the ever-vulnerable knee, the Achilles tendon and the calf muscles. Ligaments and tendons are the strongest and weakest muscles, respectively. Preventive massage plays an essential role in injury prevention and maintenance, as we will see in chapter 6. Five to ten minutes of work in this area is adequate.

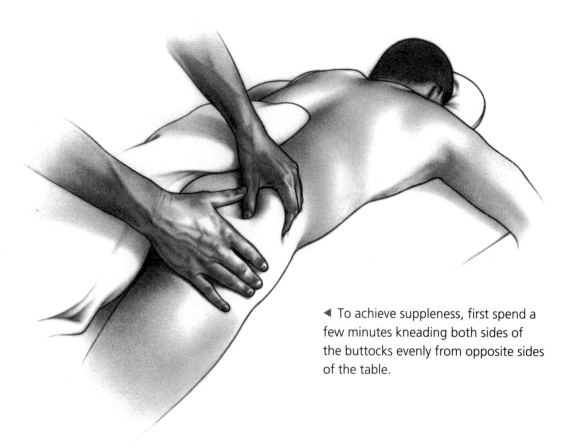

◀ To achieve suppleness, first spend a few minutes kneading both sides of the buttocks evenly from opposite sides of the table.

▼ Next, use your thumbs from the top of the buttocks to where the hamstrings attach near the bottom to work the muscles more closely.

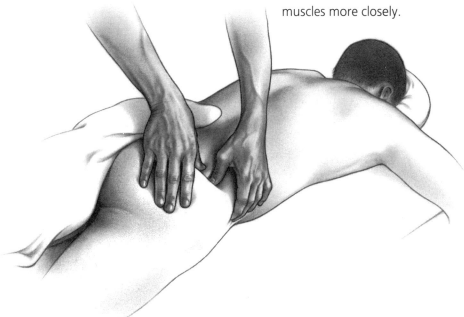

▼ To achieve a deep stroke, use your elbow. Work from the top of the buttocks down to the hamstrings.

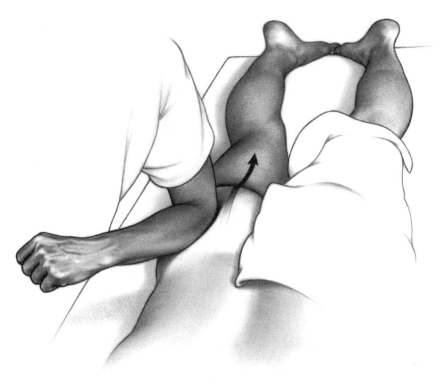

THE HAMSTRINGS

Now you're ready to spend 10 to 15 minutes concentrating on the hamstring area, though you can continue to work "through" the buttocks to reach them. Remember, everything is interconnected.

▶ First, take uncomfortable pressure off the knees by placing a pillow under the shins. Knead the hamstrings for a few minutes.

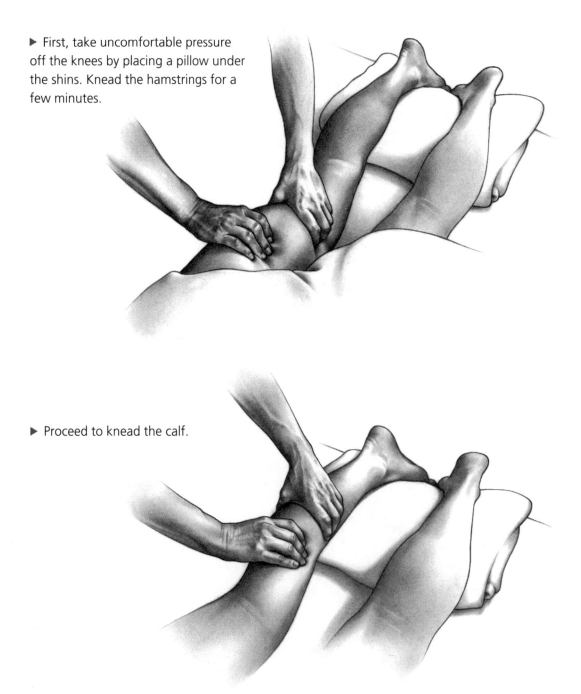

▶ Proceed to knead the calf.

▶ Close with full-length strokes from the toes to the lower back in an effleurage style. This area is now warmed up for more detailed work.

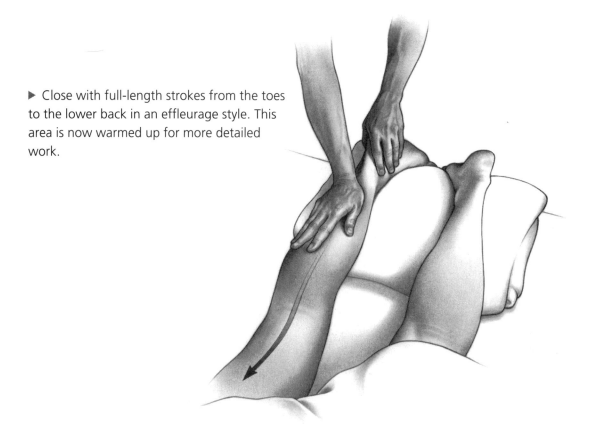

▼ Make sure the ankle and knee are supported with a pillow. Imagine the hamstring divided into four or five longitudinal strips and pick out one strip to begin to work on. Use a deep-tissue stroke up the inside of the hamstring from the knee to the buttocks, using either the palm or the knuckles. You can use the other hand to further stabilize the knee. Repeat for the other sections of the hamstrings.

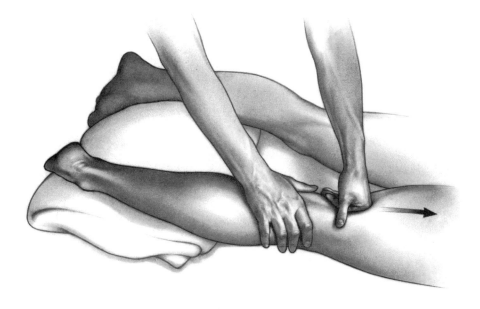

▼ Alternately, you can use both thumbs running up the leg in a similar fashion. Be sure to ease up on the tendon running on the very outside of the leg. *Important*: Do not put any direct pressure on the back of the knee.

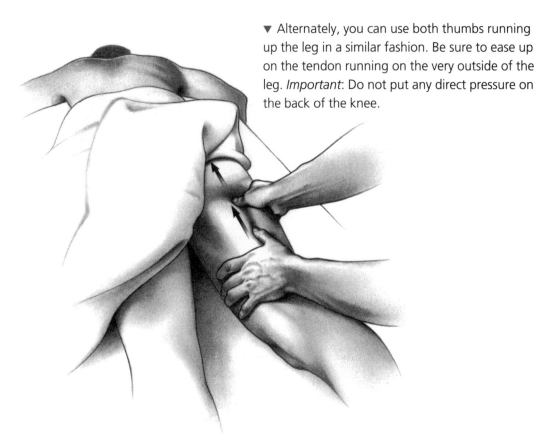

▶ Next comes a broad cross-fiber stroking on the hamstrings. Using the thumb, cross the muscles of the upper leg at 90-degree angles. Apply deep cross-fiber strokes, rubbing back and forth across the grain of the muscle with the fingertips without allowing your fingers to slide across the skin. Devote extra time and attention to tight or sore areas. Work especially the middle group as it joins the buttocks. You will find that these will be slow strokes working the breadth of one muscle at a time.

▶ Now turn your attention to the lower leg—the calf. Knead the calf again to warm this area up.

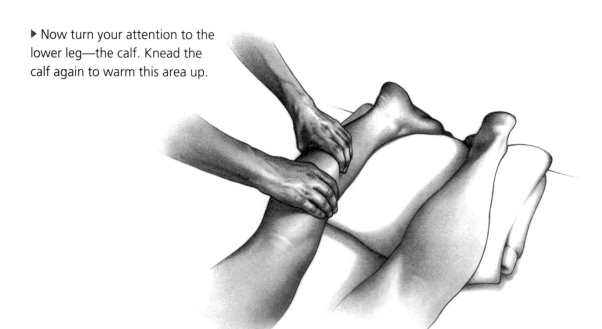

▶ Use full-length strokes from toes to lower back in an effleurage style, as you did earlier.

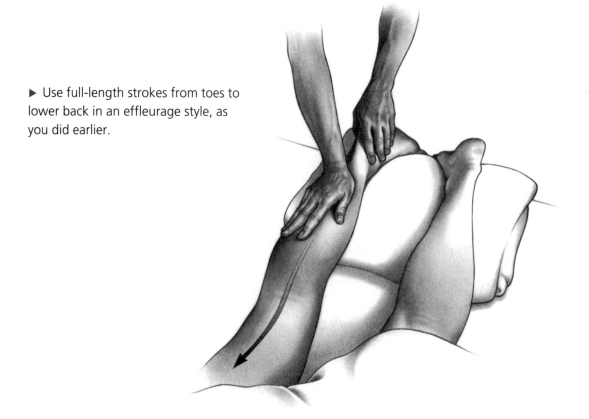

▼ Use your thumbs, joined, starting at the base of the ankle where the Achilles tendon merges into the calf. Using moderate pressure, run your thumbs up to the back of the knee but not into the knee. First go up the middle and then on either side. Repeat this three times.

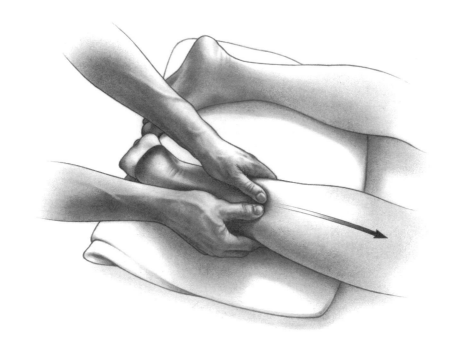

▼ Next, use a deep cross-fiber technique as you would on the hamstring. Concentrate on the belly, or fullest part, of the calf muscle. Be ever so careful of the pressure along the Achilles tendon and, of course, the back of the knee and knee joint.

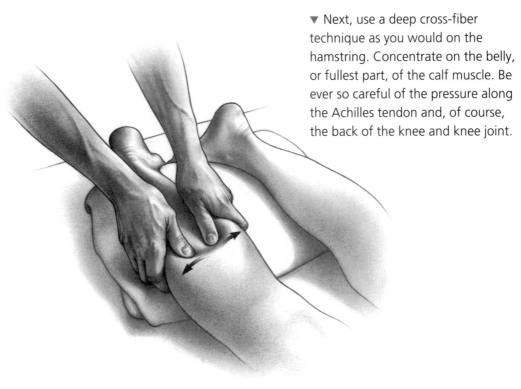

THE ANKLES

In many massage books, the ankles are a forgotten connection between the leg and foot. This joint, like any other, holds tension and needs care, too! This is true for all athletes who primarily use their lower bodies but particularly for those who do pounding, weight-bearing activities such as running. If you suffer from stiff ankles, you may have poor circulation to your feet—which massage can help improve. So working this area is invaluable!

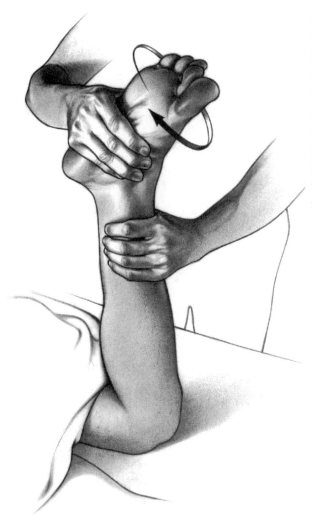

◄ Rotating the ankle will give you a sense of your friend's flexibility in this area. First, rotate the ankle to warm it up. Begin by holding the ankle with one hand, grasping the foot with the other hand and slowly moving it clockwise, then counterclockwise, in small circles and proceeding to slightly larger circles. Circle the foot to its natural limits. Repeat three times in each direction.

▼ Next, flex the foot by pushing down and then pulling up.

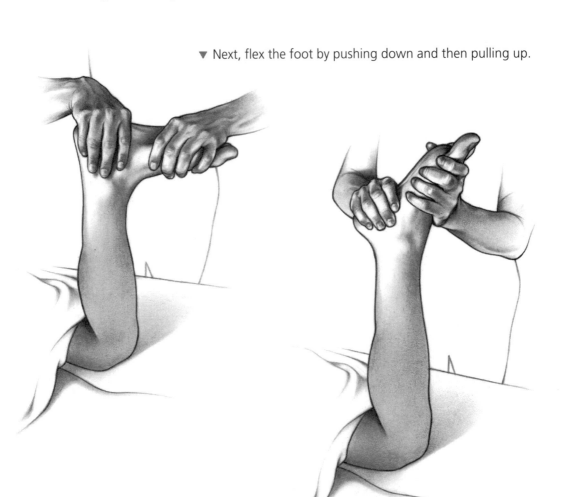

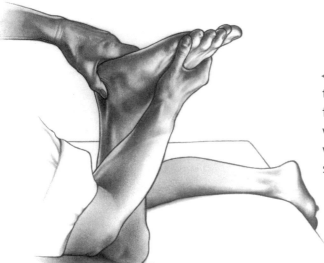

◀ Proceed to work the finer muscles and tendons around the ankle with your fingers and thumbs. Hold the foot firmly with one hand and use the other hand to work around the anklebone on both sides of the ankle.

THE FEET

The foot is the foundation of the body. This highly complex structure contains 26 small bones, which carry the entire weight of our bodies. Not only are your feet wonderful shock absorbers, they also contain thousands of nerve endings that correspond to all parts of your body internally and externally. Each muscle, organ and gland has nerves that are anchored in the feet. Thus, you are stimulating all points of the body, not just the feet themselves. Reflexologists believe that pressure on specific points of the feet will treat specific areas of the body.

Foot massage requires little lubrication; whatever lubricant is left on your hands after massaging the leg is adequate. You'll massage the feet from both the facedown position and, once your friend turns over, the faceup position, so front-of-the-foot techniques appear later in this sequence.

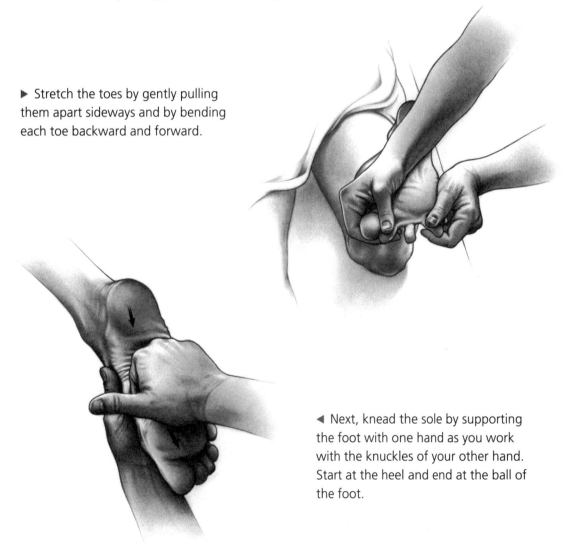

▶ Stretch the toes by gently pulling them apart sideways and by bending each toe backward and forward.

◀ Next, knead the sole by supporting the foot with one hand as you work with the knuckles of your other hand. Start at the heel and end at the ball of the foot.

▼ Now you can use your thumb to make small, circling strokes, supporting the foot with one hand as in the previous step. You can achieve much fine-detail work with this technique. Then ask if there is any other specific area that needs a little more attention. (After I've finished the entire massage, I like to ask if the body feels evenly and equally treated on both sides.) This ends the massage on the back side.

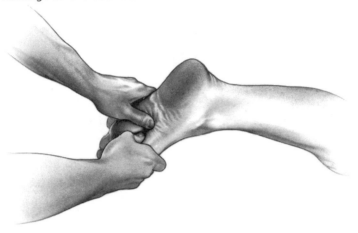

THE FRONTS OF THE LEGS

Ask your friend to turn over—"Flip like a fish," I sometimes say. Check with your friend before proceeding to see if you should put a pillow under the knees or under the neck. And check to make sure that the temperature is comfortable. I like to cover the leg that is not being worked on with an extra towel.

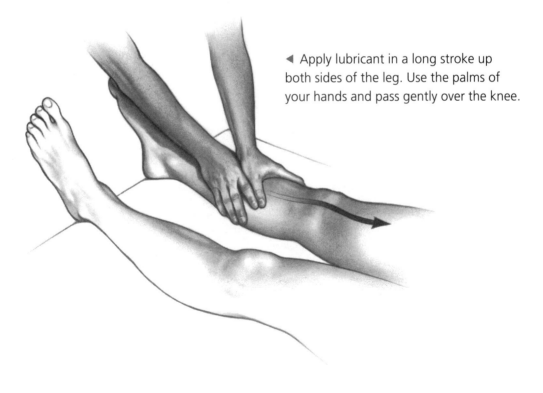

◄ Apply lubricant in a long stroke up both sides of the leg. Use the palms of your hands and pass gently over the knee.

▼ Use a long stroke up the shin—but not on the bone itself—pulling the muscle gently away from the bone. Be gentle: Athletes whose sports require a lot of lower-leg movement often have some tenderness at the top of the lower leg near the knee.

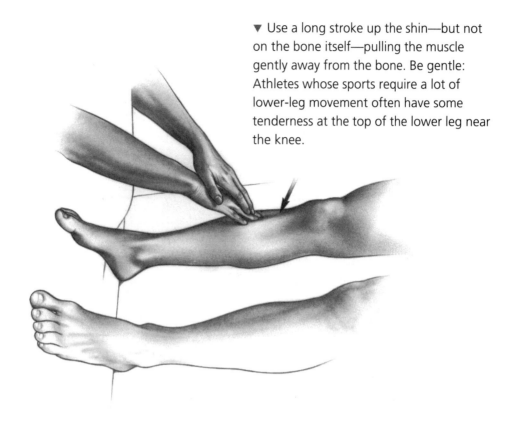

▼ Next, shake, squeeze and knead to loosen and relax the quads. Place your hands on the outside of the thigh and roll the quads between them. Repeat on the other leg. Ten or 15 minutes here is fine.

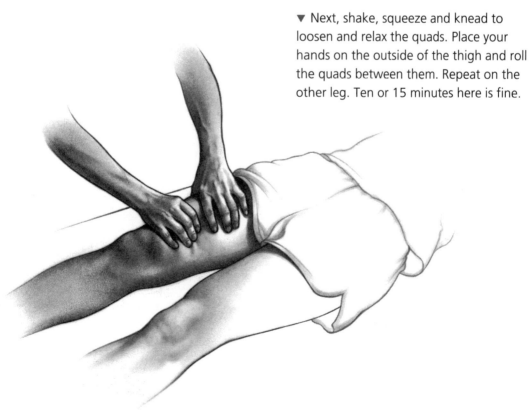

▼ With the fronts of the legs warmed up, let's get more specific. The strokes you use here are similar to the ones on the back of the leg; however, the anatomy is different—you'll be working near the bony areas of the shin and knee. Use the V of your hand between the thumbs and fingers and press firmly upward along both sides of the shinbone. Use both hands alternately, moving from the ankle to the knee. Feel the fleshy parts on either side of the shinbone—this is an area where athletes sometimes report having the painful condition known as shinsplints. Preventive massage here can eliminate much of the tightness associated with this common condition. Be careful not to apply direct pressure on top of the bone. Repeat this up to six times.

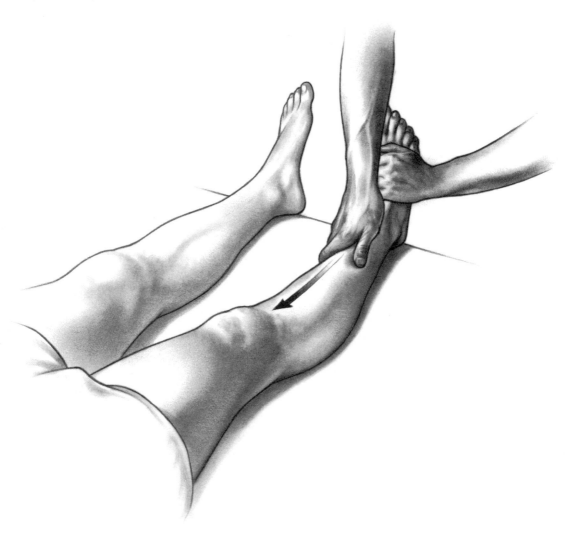

▼ Next, make the outside shin muscles more accessible by turning the foot in slightly. Using a firmer and deeper stroke, join both thumbs as you move slowly from the ankle to the base of the knee joint. This is where the muscle attaches, and by working this area thoroughly you can restore its length and suppleness. Any push-off movement required in athletic activity will now seem more powerful and fluid.

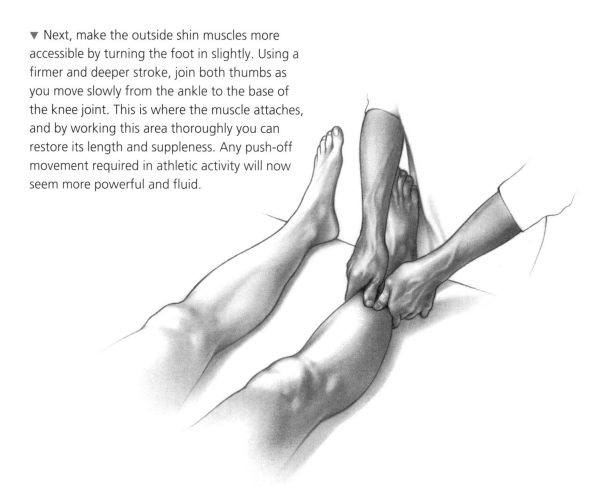

▼ Now apply gentle traction to the lower leg by pulling on the foot with both hands. Repeat three times.

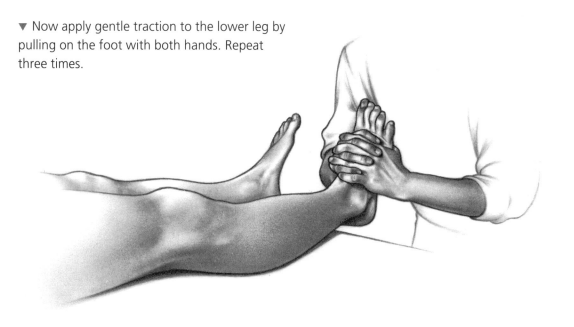

THE KNEES

Healthy knees are vital to an active life. Three long bones meet at the knee joint: the femur of the thigh and the tibia and fibula of the lower leg. The patella, popularly known as the kneecap, protects this joint, yet it remains one of the most vulnerable parts of the human body. The knee is held together by a sensitive and complex combination of ligaments, and the muscles of the lower and upper leg all meet here.

Without underestimating this area, preventive massage can reduce tension, restore length and suppleness and reduce the likelihood of injury from the many sports that make rigorous demands on the legs and knees.

▶ Using the heels of your hands, apply pressure around the knee by moving from the base and top to the outside in a circle.

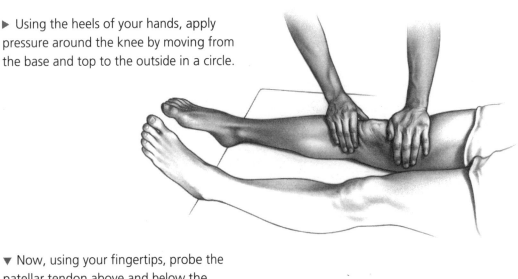

▼ Now, using your fingertips, probe the patellar tendon above and below the kneecap as shown. If there is any pain, see a sports medicine professional. If not, clasp one hand behind the knee and use the fingertips of the other hand to make small circles around the knee.

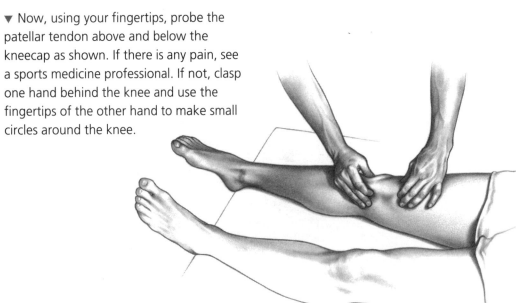

THE QUADS

You are now ready to work the large muscles of the quadriceps.

▼ Standing or sitting at the side of your
friend near the knee, you can again knead
the quad to warm it up for deeper work.

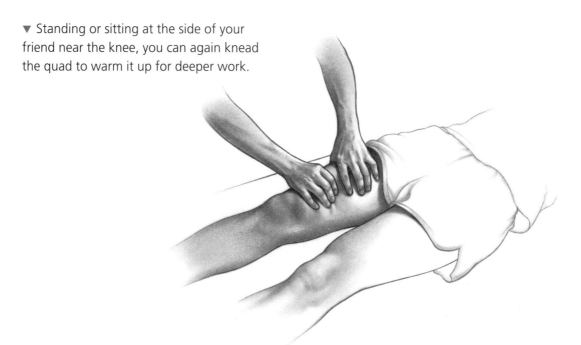

▼ As with the hamstrings, visually divide the quads into four parts. Begin by working the
outside of this group along the iliotibial band. This long tendon runs from the upper crest of
the hip and attaches below the outside of the knee on the major bone of the lower leg.
Many athletes know when this is tight. Use a cross-fiber stroke that is moderate in pressure.
Then use your palm to apply effleurage from the outside of the knee to the top of the
hipbone (also known as the pelvis). Repeat this three times, then repeat for the second, third
and fourth sections of the quads.

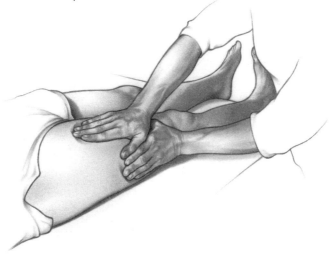

▶ With your thumbs joined, as shown, cover each one of those four sections, using as deep a pressure as your friend can comfortably tolerate. For each section, start at the top of the knee and follow through until you reach the hip.

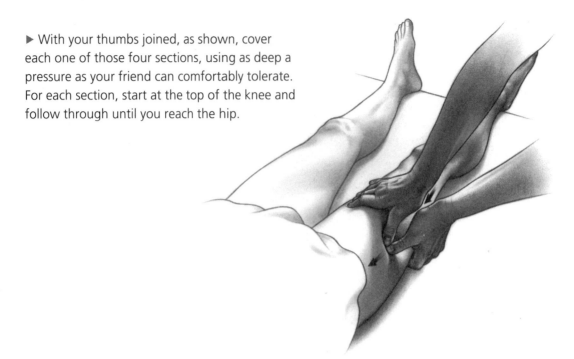

▼ I like to finish off the leg by returning to the full-length stroke shown below. Repeat three times. At the finish, try gently pulling the leg by cupping one hand around your friend's heel and the other on top of the foot. Raise the foot a few inches off the table or ground and, as you lean back, pull the leg gently; release and repeat. This feels great on all three joints—the hip, knee and ankle. If there has been any surgery on any of these joints, consult a sports medicine expert before attempting this. Make sure the grip is comfortable for your friend and remember to lean with your body weight and not just the arms.

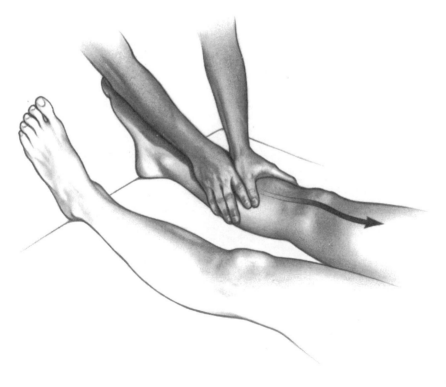

THE FEET

Preventive massage on the feet keeps them healthy. I have found that injuries that start in this intricate and complex structure inevitably move up the leg, manifesting themselves in other injuries. By spotting little aches and pains early, you can keep your training injury-free!

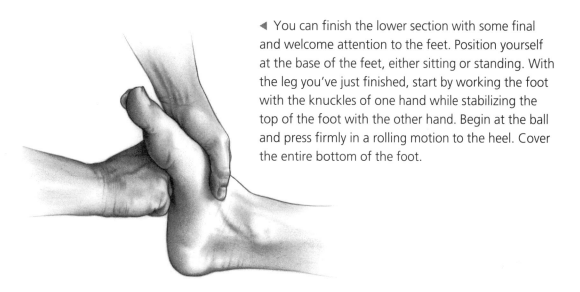

◄ You can finish the lower section with some final and welcome attention to the feet. Position yourself at the base of the feet, either sitting or standing. With the leg you've just finished, start by working the foot with the knuckles of one hand while stabilizing the top of the foot with the other hand. Begin at the ball and press firmly in a rolling motion to the heel. Cover the entire bottom of the foot.

► Next, "open" the foot by sliding the heels of your hands from the middle top of the foot to its outside. Work from the ball of the foot to the ankle. This is really a stretch across the top of the foot and benefits its complex structure by opening up these intricate spaces, spreading out compressed fascia, tendons and muscles.

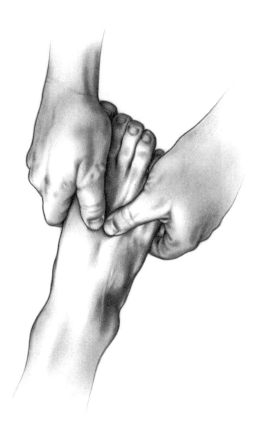

◀ Now use your thumbs in small strokes on the tops and bottoms of the feet. Start on the top and use firm pressure to follow the valleys and tendons. Be detailed and thorough. Work around the toes and ankles as well.

▶ Pull each toe with gentle traction, starting with the big toe.

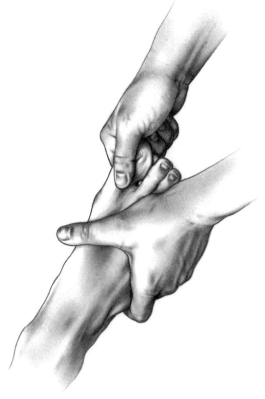

▼ Next, go to the bottom of the foot and work slowly and thoroughly. If you are working on a table, you may find it relaxing to sit in a chair at the base of the table as you spend your time on this area. If you are working on the ground, prop your friend's feet up into your lap or use a pillow for easier access and comfort. Spend some added time working the arches of the feet using deep strokes. Work for ten minutes on the feet if this is part of a full-body massage. Stabilize the ankle with one hand and work deeply with the thumb of the other.

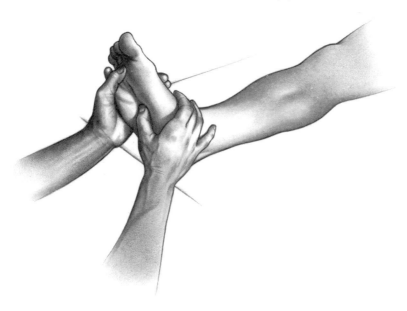

▼ I like to end this section by again gently pulling the leg as mentioned on page 58. As the giver, center yourself by focusing on your breathing as you clasp one foot with both hands while applying gentle traction. Repeat the same sequence on the other foot. Before moving on, do a little courtesy—cover the lower half of your friend with a blanket or a couple of towels. This provides a sense of comfort and security.

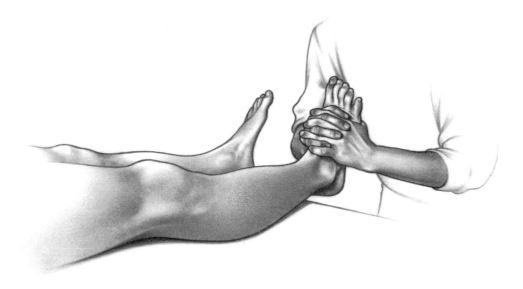

THE FRONT OF THE TORSO

The chest and abdomen are sensitive areas. This part of our body reflects the way we feel about ourselves and how we face the world. The torso consists of the rib cage, which contains the heart, lungs and various other organs, and the abdomen, which contains some of our deepest feelings. Your stomach can churn when you're tense; your heart can beat madly when you're embarrassed; your lungs can work busily to supply air when you're frightened or exhilarated. So be aware of the emotional vulnerability of the person you're massaging. Some women are also modest about their breasts, so I drape this area differently for males and females. For males, I leave the torso exposed; for females, I drape the chest with a towel. Either way, first ask the person you're massaging about this. By establishing boundaries, you gain the recipient's respect and trust.

On a personal note, it has taken me years to feel comfortable both as a giver and as a receiver. Massage therapy has given me a gift of body awareness just as sport has!

The chest is a maze of muscles with an amazing number of tendon attachments all along the rib cage and along the spine and shoulder blades. Upper-body sports such as tennis, rock climbing, wrestling and others demand much from these areas.

You can knead the upper chest as you would any other large muscle mass. In my opinion, however, working the finer intercostal muscles—the ones between the ribs—should be left to a professional sports therapist. Likewise, on a superficial level, the muscles of the abdomen can be massaged safely. Deep massage in these areas, however, is best left to the professional sports therapist.

▶ (Top of page 63) So, let's start with the chest. Stand or kneel above your friend's head. With your hands well-oiled, glide your hands over the torso, covering the surface of the chest and abdomen. Rest your hands gently in the middle of the upper chest just below the collarbone. Use the entire surface of the hands, with the fingers pointing toward the feet and thumbs touching each other. Use firm pressure as you start and ease up as you reach the stomach. Use a long stroke down the center to the navel and sweep your hands wide as you pull back up along the sides. On women, these strokes should move around the breasts.

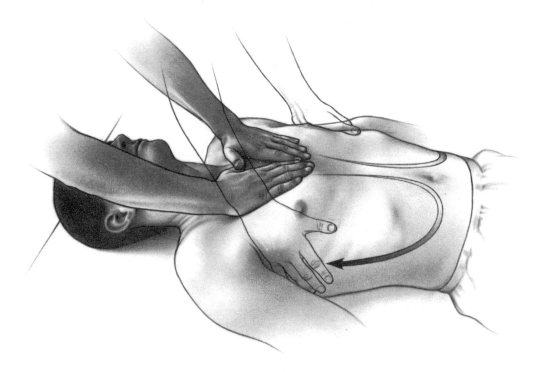

▼ Stand or kneel on either side of your friend at the waist. Using the fingertips of both hands, gently stroke the abdomen in a clockwise direction. This should be a gliding movement. In this manner you follow the path of digestion. Make a dozen or so slow circles.

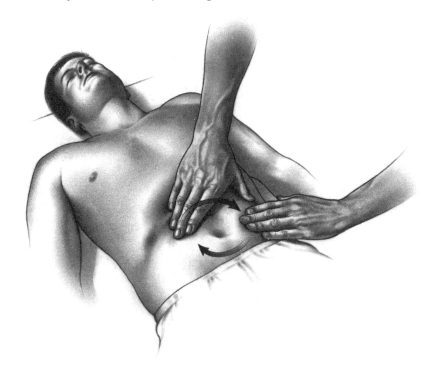

▼ I like to end this section by pulling up on the sides of the torso from the waist to the armpit. Lean across and pull up slowly yet firmly on the opposite side, with your hands alternating as you fall into a relaxed rhythm. Start at the waistline or the crest of the hipbone and travel to the armpit. Repeat this three times and then move to the other side. You will find that you can place your fingertips under the back before you begin the pulling action.

You can now cover the torso with a spare towel or extend the blanket you've used to cover the legs. Again, this gives your friend a wonderful sense of security and well-being. Leave the arms and hands exposed as we move on to this area.

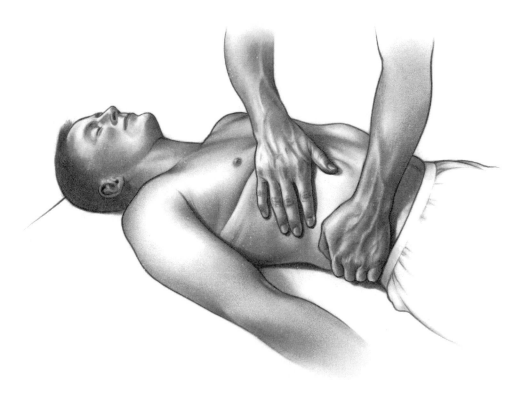

THE ARMS AND HANDS

Our arms and hands are the most active parts of our bodies in work or play. They contain major muscles, as in the upper arm, and intricate ones, as in the forearms and hands. We freely express ourselves through powerful emotions as we relate to the world around us with these instruments. Moreover, with preventive massage, most common injuries here can be minimized. A hand-and-arm massage also can relax us and help settle our tensions, anxieties and bottled-up feelings from our participation in both our daily lives and sporting lifestyles.

▼ Start on either side. Stand or kneel at your friend's side near the hand. Begin by lubricating the hand and arm using a long stroke. Start slowly, as your friend is reawakening to this part of the body. With the palm and arm flat against the surface, stabilize the wrist with one hand. Proceed to glide the other hand firmly up the arm, gently passing over the elbow, to reach the shoulder.

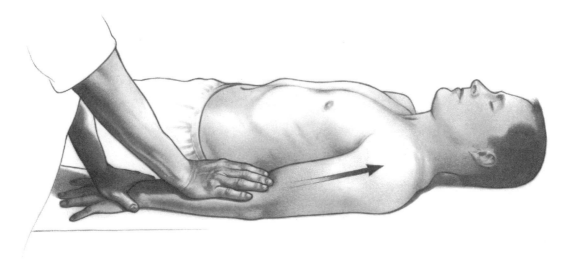

▼ When you reach the shoulder, cup this joint with your hand. Return in a fluid motion to the wrist, using both of your hands; apply a gentle pulling motion by clasping the wrist. Repeat three times.

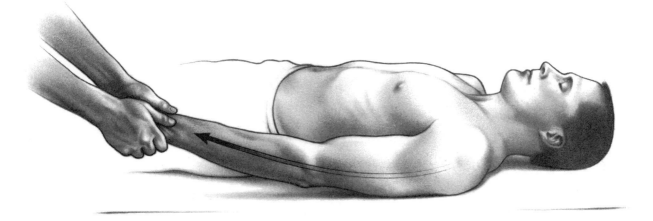

▼ Next, knead the arm as it lies flat on the surface. Move from the wrist to the shoulder and then back down again. After you've kneaded the arm three times, repeat the previous stroke once.

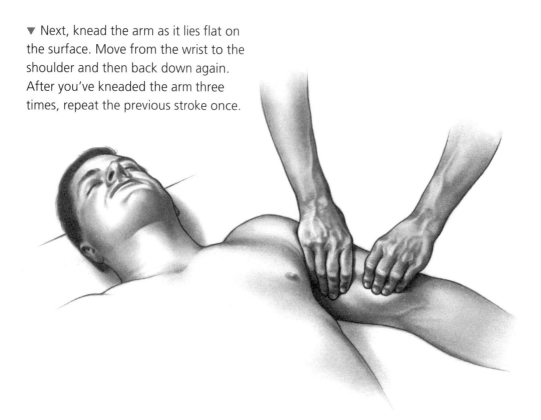

▼ This stroke is referred to as milking or draining the arm. Lift your friend's forearm off the table. Make a ring around the wrist with the fingers and thumbs of both hands, with both thumbs touching against the inside of the wrist. Slide both hands down with firm pressure all the way to the elbow; return to the wrist with your hands loose, remaining in contact with the skin but not applying pressure. Repeat this three to six times, exploring pressure and speed.

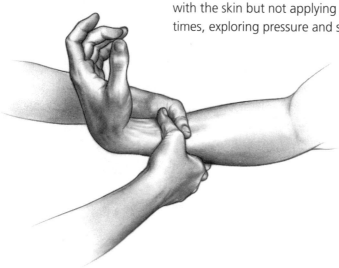

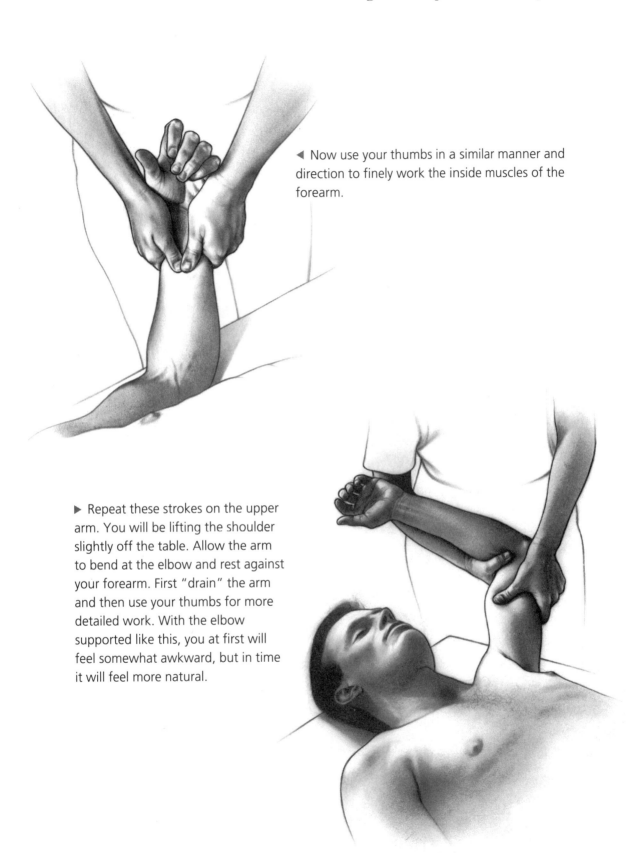

◄ Now use your thumbs in a similar manner and direction to finely work the inside muscles of the forearm.

▶ Repeat these strokes on the upper arm. You will be lifting the shoulder slightly off the table. Allow the arm to bend at the elbow and rest against your forearm. First "drain" the arm and then use your thumbs for more detailed work. With the elbow supported like this, you at first will feel somewhat awkward, but in time it will feel more natural.

▼ Clasping your friend's hand in your own, work the finer muscles of the outside of the forearm with your thumbs as the arm remains on the table or floor. Again, move from the wrist to the elbow. Start up the middle and then proceed to the sides. As you near the elbow you will likely find tender spots, as almost everyone has them. Next, move to the upper arm and brace it with one hand at the elbow. Use a similar stroke with your thumbs as you separate the biceps from the triceps.

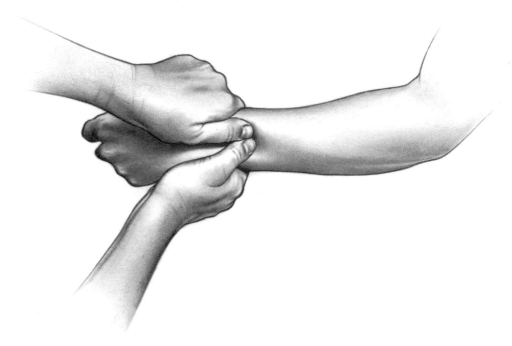

▼ Proceed to the hand and do some gentle pulling of the fingers and thumbs.

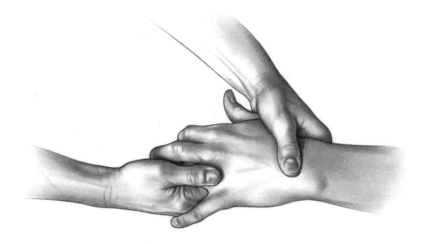

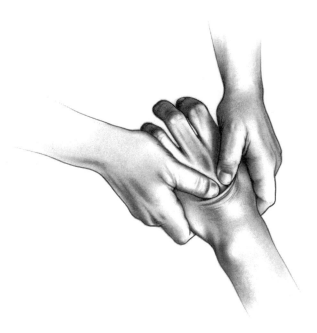

◄ As you gently hold the hand to be massaged, work with your thumbs around the inside and outside of the hand. The detailed work here is similar to that on the feet. Then work the tendons on the back of the hand as you would the top of the feet, all the way around the wrist.

▼ End this section by again pulling on the arm as you gradually lean back with your body. You can add variety by pulling down, across and over the shoulder. Repeat this sequence on the other arm.

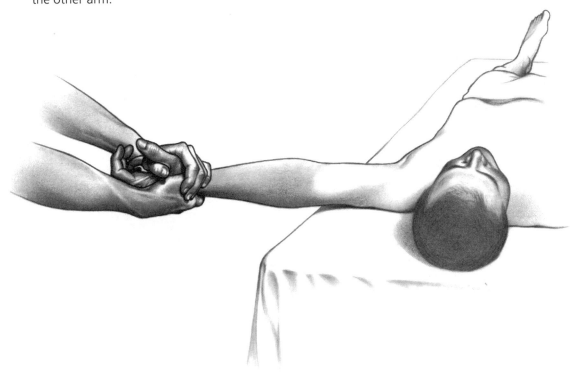

THE NECK AND HEAD

Massaging the neck and head is a great way to end a massage—or as a session by itself. It is almost always a high-tension area. Think about the stress you read in people's faces every day. Massage is a welcome way to soothe away this tension.

▼ Begin by applying gentle stretches to the neck. Hold the base of the skull in your hands and lift the head a little off the surface. Pull gently toward you. Repeat this three times.

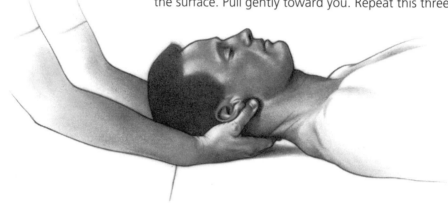

◀ Next, bring the chin to the chest by gently lifting the head off the table or surface. Release slowly and repeat. Now, ever so gently move the head from side to side.

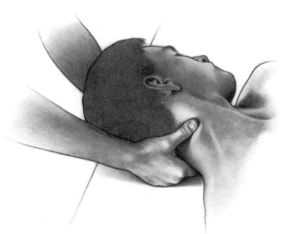

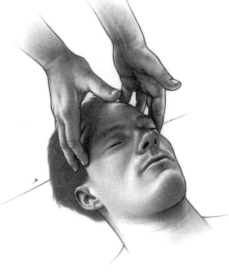

▶ Slowly place the head back on the surface to begin a scalp and facial massage. Make sure the head is aligned naturally with the spine. There should be no flexion or extension of the neck, head and shoulders.

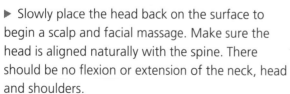

▼ As you move to the face, you will need no additional lubricant. Start by massaging the whole scalp with your fingers. Tug the hair gently; most people love this.

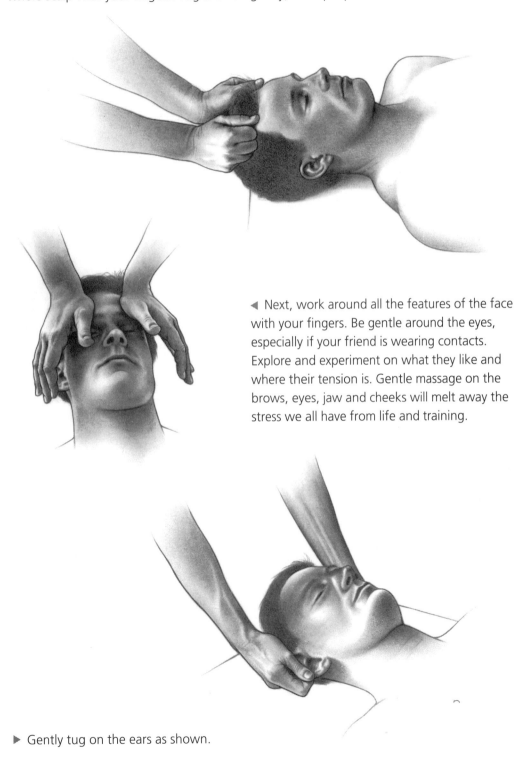

◄ Next, work around all the features of the face with your fingers. Be gentle around the eyes, especially if your friend is wearing contacts. Explore and experiment on what they like and where their tension is. Gentle massage on the brows, eyes, jaw and cheeks will melt away the stress we all have from life and training.

▶ Gently tug on the ears as shown.

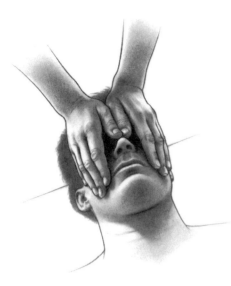

◀ You have now completed a full-body massage. Slowly warm your hands by rubbing them together to generate heat and then place them over your friend's eyes for several moments. This is a wonderful way to end a session with the person feeling whole. A deep sense of relaxation enables us to reconnect.

▼ A final word: Gently give your friend a short verbal indicator that you are finished. Place an additional blanket over the body. Leave the space your friend is relaxing in; you should always allow the person you're massaging to rise at a comfortable pace. You don't want to put an abrupt halt to the sense of peace and relaxation that has resulted from the massage.

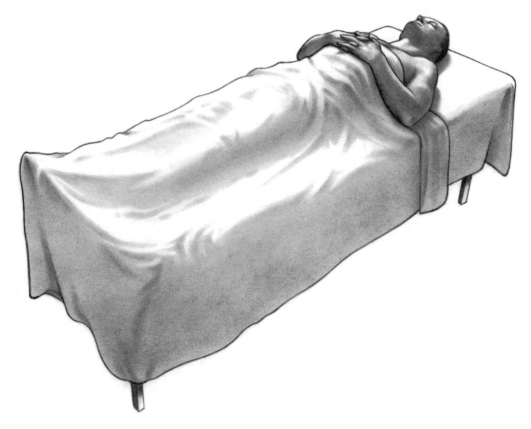

How to Find (or Become) a Sports Massage Therapist

Massage is a science as well as a healing art, and a good therapist integrates scientific knowledge with technical skills, sensitivity and awareness. While everyone has the ability to learn massage, it takes a solid training process to become a professional practitioner.

Finding a massage therapist. To locate a professional sports massage therapist, you can contact the American Massage Therapy Association (AMTA), 820 Davis Street, Evanston, IL 60201; (708) 864-0123.

In addition, ask your friends, co-workers and/or sports medicine professionals for their referrals. You can also look in the Yellow Pages under "Massage" or in local sports publications under "Services."

Ask the therapist (or therapists) you are considering about their training, approach, certification and fees. Ask for references. This initial conversation is a good time to begin assessing how your personalities mesh—or don't. Don't be afraid to discuss any apprehensions or concerns. Trust is important; you should feel confident and comfortable with your therapist.

Locating a massage school. I went to massage school after getting an undergraduate degree in sports science from Iowa State University. Never in my wildest dreams did I think I'd make a living as a massage therapist. That was over a decade ago, and I simply wanted to learn more. Now I love what I do and would never trade in this rewarding experience.

If at some point you feel that you'd like to pursue a career in sports massage therapy, the best schools are approved by the AMTA. These schools offer programs consisting of at least 500 hours of training. Check with your city and state for licensing and certification requirements if you are thinking of a career move. Check with the school you are interested in for length, content and cost of their program. The school can help answer questions pertaining to the requirements to practice.

5

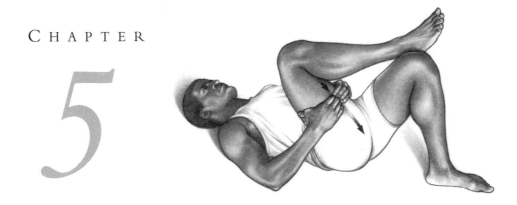

SELF-MASSAGE TECHNIQUES

Know thyself.

INSCRIPTION AT THE DELPHIC ORACLE, FROM *Plutarch's Morals*

You may never be able to achieve the massage therapist's leverage, depth or vigorousness during self-massage. But one day you may find yourself in need of massage with no one's hands available but your own. That is the time to get a grip on yourself—literally.

Your body is an amazing machine. But like any machine, it needs the occasional tune-up to keep it running smoothly. If you're dragging, self-massage can restore your snap. If you're stressed from intense exercise, it can cut recovery time dramatically. With regular applications of self-massage, you'll find yourself looking and feeling better. For these reasons, self-massage should be an integral part of every athlete's training program.

A healthy awareness of your body has its own psychological rewards. Learning hands-on, therapeutic touch allows you to discover what feels good and what doesn't in massage, what needs work, and what problems might be lurking just below the skin. Self-massage gives you an opportunity to explore your own physiology while getting direct, instantaneous biofeedback. By learning and practicing the following self-massage techniques, you will increase your body's ability to perform and recover.

MASSAGING THE PARTS YOU CAN REACH

Lie on your back in a comfortable position with a pillow under your knees and calves. Relax your entire body, including your face, jaw, extremities and torso. Breathe slowly and deeply. After relaxing for several minutes, begin with the following self-massages.

HANDS

▶ Manipulate areas of discomfort with the thumb and fingers of the massaging hand. Apply firm but gentle direct pressure to sore or tender areas. Massage the palm by interlocking your fingers and then working the surface of the palm by supplying direct pressure or stroking with the thumb.

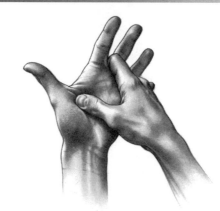

FEET

▶ While seated, rest one foot on the opposite thigh. Use your thumbs, fingers and palms to massage up and down the bottom of the foot. Concentrate on the arch. Stroke lengthwise or try circular motions. Pull and separate the toes.

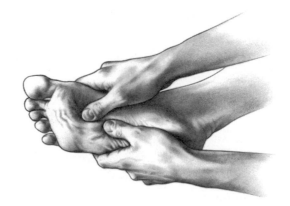

CALVES

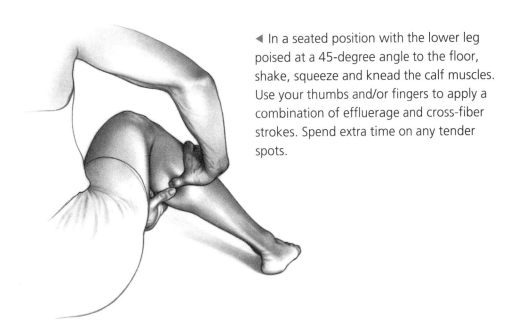

◀ In a seated position with the lower leg poised at a 45-degree angle to the floor, shake, squeeze and knead the calf muscles. Use your thumbs and/or fingers to apply a combination of effluerage and cross-fiber strokes. Spend extra time on any tender spots.

SHINS

▶ Press your thumbs into the muscle near your ankle and stroke up the leg toward the knee as shown. Another good shin massage is to loosen and relax the muscles of the shin using your thumbs and fingertips. Starting out lightly and applying more pressure, use slower cross-fiber strokes. Concentrate on tight or tender areas, especially the upper part of the muscle.

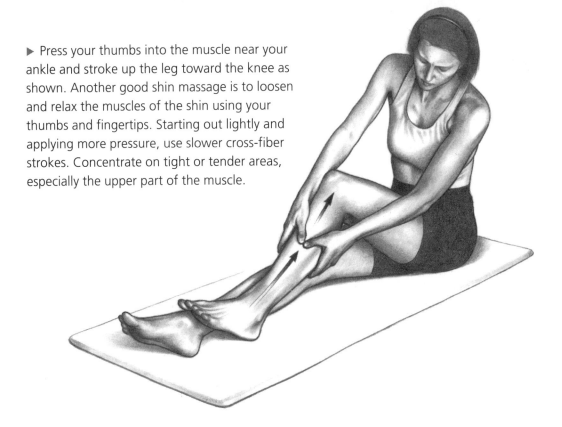

QUADRICEPS

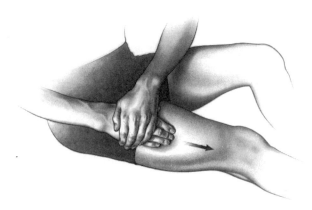

◀ Massage the outside of the quads, holding your middle three fingers together with the middle finger bent slightly. Press one hand on top of the other to help control the stroke. Push your fingers along your leg to just above your knee. You can also do this massage for your adductors, on the inside of your legs.

▶ Loosen and relax the quads by shaking, squeezing and kneading. Vigorously roll the quad back and forth between your hands. Visually divide the muscle into longitudinal sections, using your thumbs and fingers to perform cross-fiber strokes. Then press your thumbs into the muscle on the top of the leg and push your thumbs downward toward the knee.

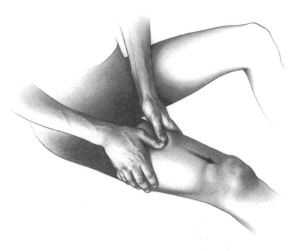

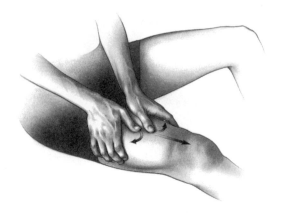

◀ Move your thumbs in a circular fashion, alternating thumbs and moving your hands toward the knee.

HAMSTRINGS

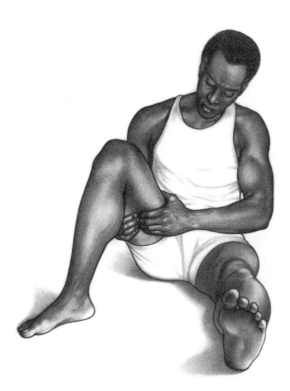

◀ Placing your foot flat on the floor, sit comfortably against a wall with your back supported. As you bend your knee, this position relaxes the leg, making it easier for you to work on it. Use one or both hands to shake, squeeze and knead the hamstrings, working the entire length of the muscle.

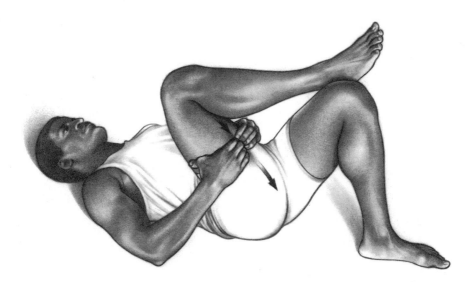

▲ While lying flat on your back, press the tips of your fingers into your hamstrings so the backs of the fingers of one hand are in contact with the backs of the fingers of the other hand. Press firmly into the muscle and move your fingers down toward the buttocks.

BUTTOCKS

▼ With your thigh raised close to your chest, use the fingertips of your outside hand to press deeply against the "sit bone." Press deeply with a cross-fiber technique. Pain in this area may indicate inflammation of the tendon. Consult a sports therapist if it persists.

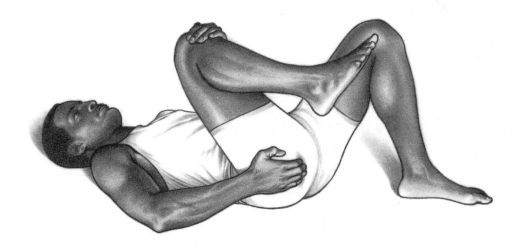

LOWER BACK

▼ Lie on a tennis ball, with the ball directly under the area you want to massage and with as much of your body weight on the ball as is comfortable. You can also use this technique for massaging the buttocks.

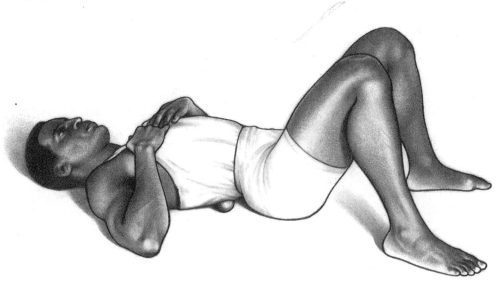

ARMS

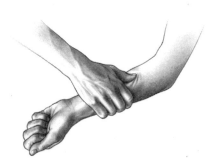

◄ Massage muscles of the posterior forearm by stroking the arm, both palm down and palm up, with your thumb. The muscles of the anterior surface of the forearm may be loosened by pressing on trigger points on the forearm while alternately clenching and opening the fist.

► You can reach the triceps by placing your arm in front of your body with the elbow bent at a 90-degree angle. Work down toward the elbow with the fingertips while slowly straightening the arm. Be gentle with the area just above your elbow where the triceps muscles converge at the triceps tendon.

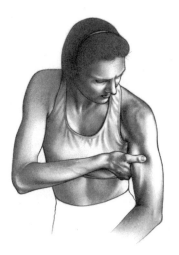

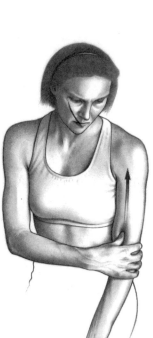

◄ Massage the biceps by stroking longitudinally from the elbow toward the armpit with the thumb. Continue to the upper biceps, pressing the thumb transversely into the junction of the biceps muscles. Continue upward onto the anterior deltoid with the thumb. Press firmly along the length of the biceps tendon, with each stroke finishing at the top of the shoulder.

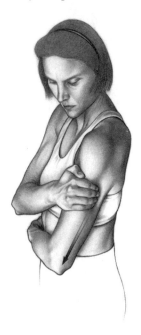

► Grip the inside of the arm as shown. Press lightly into the tendon (this is the junction of the biceps) and rock it back and forth.

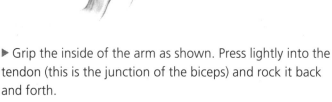

CHEST

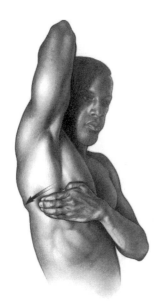

▼ This massage works your pectoralis major and minor. Hold your middle three fingers tightly together, with the middle finger slightly bent so those three fingers almost form a line. Press into the muscle close to the sternum and stroke from the sternum to the shoulder with the tips of the fingers. Place the hand on the side being massaged behind your head to offer a gentle stretch.

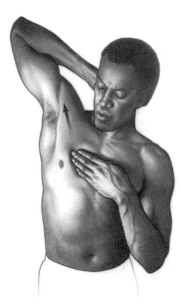

▲ This works the latissimus dorsi muscle of the chest. Work downward or across the entire muscle. Use short strokes and maintain constant pressure with the fingertips.

NECK

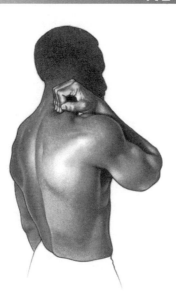

◄ Press your fingers firmly into the trapezius muscle, from just below the skull to the shoulder. Continue by tilting the head away from the hand while dragging your fingers toward the shoulder.

SHOULDERS

▶ Press the fingertips of one hand into the muscle at the top of the other shoulder. Rock your fingers backward and forward to massage the muscle.

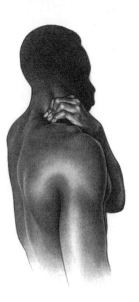

GETTING THE UNREACHABLE PARTS

What about a more thorough massage for places you can't easily reach on your own body: the back, buttocks, neck, hamstrings and shoulders? Self-massage wouldn't be of much use if you were unable to treat such vital parts of the anatomy. Bears scratch their backs against the trunks of trees, cows rub their necks on fences, and your dog does that butt-drag thing across the carpet. These animals are pretty resourceful when it comes to inventing ways to attend to the parts of their bodies that are out of reach. Luckily for us, someone out there has cleverly invented a number of simple tools that make our unreachable spots reachable without the involvement of tree bark, barbed wire or carpet fiber.

One enormously useful tool is called the Thera Cane (shown on page 89), manufactured by Pro Massage Company of Denver, Colorado. This handy device can enable you to reach trigger points or tender spots on your own when a partner isn't handy or you can't get to a sports massage therapist.

Designed by a former chronic pain sufferer to help relieve his own discomfort, the Thera Cane is made of fiberglass and allows you access to hard-to-reach areas. The manufacturer notes that it's important to keep the ball in contact with your body. Massaging across the muscle fibers while maintaining pressure is the best technique to restore circulation to knotted muscle fibers. For best results, use the Thera Cane as part of an ongoing reconditioning program that includes moist heat, ice, stretching, and strengthening exercises.

The Thera Cane comes with specific illustrated directions for use. The manufacturer suggests that overuse may cause muscle soreness and advises users to keep sessions short at first. The Thera Cane is sold at many physical therapy and medical supply stores. You can order one through Stretching, Inc., P.O. Box 767, Palmer Lake, CO 80133; 1-800-333-1307, or The Massage Store, Ltd., P.O. Box 2247, Boulder, CO 80306; 1-800-728-2426.

Roll into a Massage

You can also effectively massage yourself with a Massage Roller, a simple, inexpensive device that allows you to use your own body weight to apply pressure to many hard-to-reach spots. The roller itself consists of a six-inch section of Ethafoam cylinder, typically cut into three-foot sections for massage uses. Ethafoam cylinders are often stocked by packaging businesses; ask them to cut a three-foot section for you. Some physical therapists may also be able to sell you one, or you can order directly through Foam Roller Therapy, from The Massage Store, Ltd. (see above for address).

UPPER BACK

▼ Allow the back to arch and the chest to "open up" as you lie back on the roller to work the upper back. Avoid rolling lower than the bottom of the rib cage or higher than mid-scapula. Keep the motion small and move slowly.

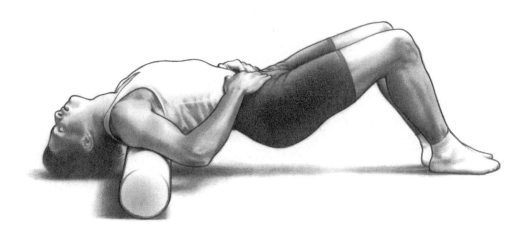

MIDDLE BACK

▼ For the middle back, maintain firm abdominal muscles and a flat back, never allowing the back to arch. Roll from mid-rib cage to lower back. Move slowly and carefully, gently rolling out the tight spots. Begin by rolling the rows of muscles on either side of the spinal column simultaneously, then proceed to emphasize one side or the other. Roll down on both rows of muscles; roll up emphasizing one side or the other.

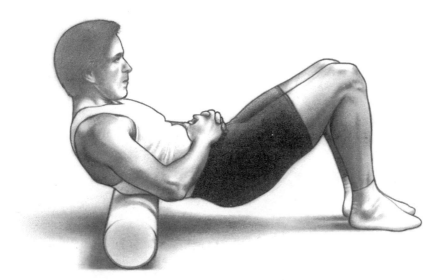

CHEST

▼ Iron out both pectorals simultaneously or individually.

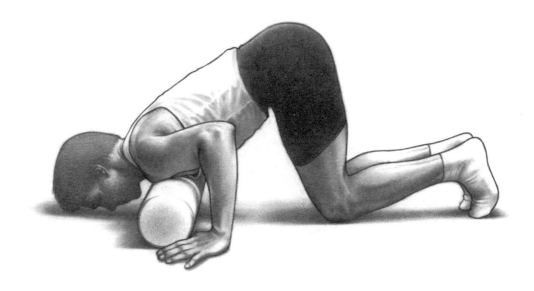

BUTTOCKS

▼ Use a very small rolling range from the center of the buttocks muscle to the top of the hipbones. Avoid rolling across the "point" of the hip onto the hamstring or beyond the hipbones onto the lower back.

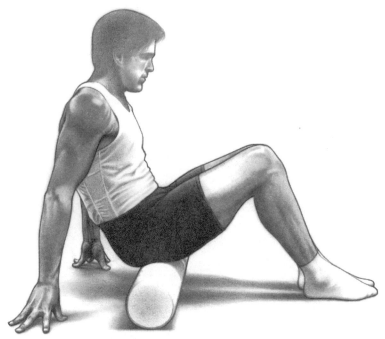

HAMSTRINGS

▼ Keeping the opposite foot flat on the floor, roll from mid-hamstring to mid-buttocks by twisting slightly as you roll. Keep the rolling leg straight and elevated.

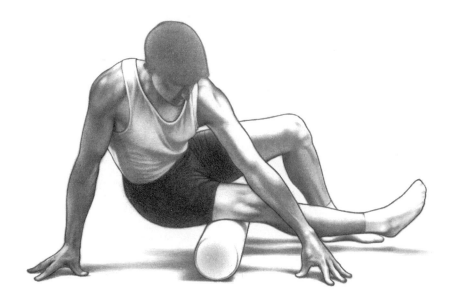

▼ Roll the length of the hamstring from above and behind the knee to the insertion of the buttocks muscle. Keep your back and legs straight, at about a 90-degree angle, and keep your legs together.

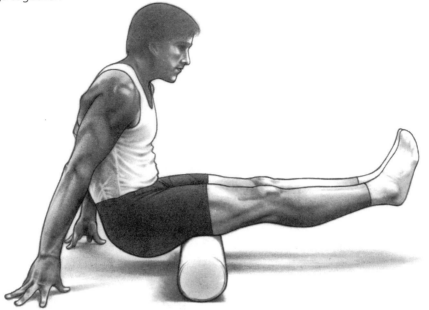

▼ With your legs open, twist to one side and roll first the inside of one thigh and the outside of the other. Then twist to the other side and repeat.

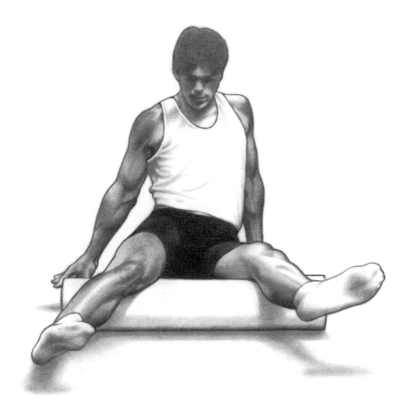

QUADRICEPS

▼ With your legs extended and relaxed, roll the quadriceps from the upper thigh to just above the knee. Experiment with rolling both legs simultaneously or one leg at a time, resting the inner thigh of the free leg on the roller.

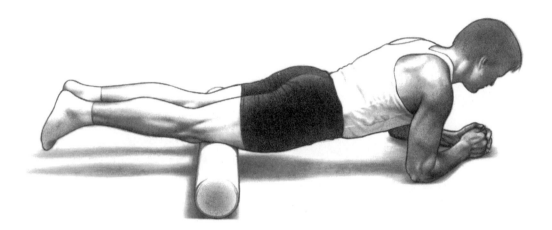

ILIOTIBIAL BAND

▼ With your weight on the lateral thigh, gently roll out the length of the iliotibial band from just above the knee to past the point of the hip. This one will hurt at first. Start slowly and keep the pressure light until it becomes more bearable. It'll get better.

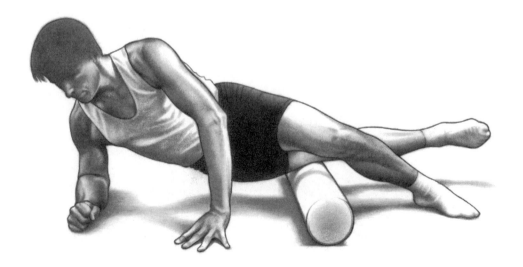

INNER THIGH

▼ Roll from knee to upper thigh, maintaining consistent pressure in both directions. Move slowly, concentrating gently on tight or tender spots. Work different angles of the inner thigh to apply pressure to the quadriceps, sartorios, groin and adductor muscles.

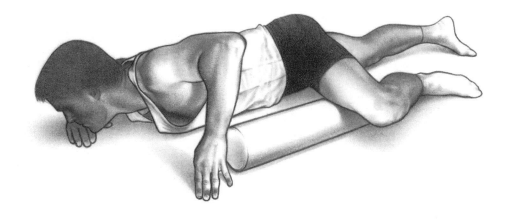

THERA CANE

▶ You can use this versatile tool to massage just about every part of your body. It comes with detailed, illustrated instructions.

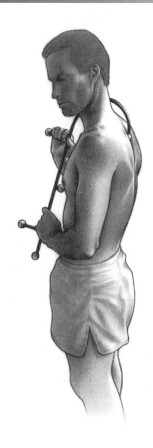

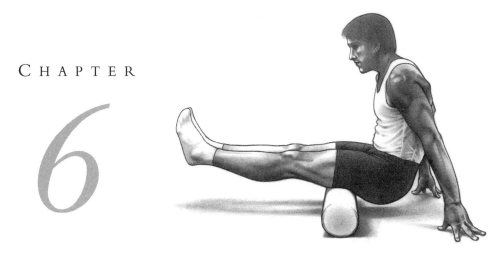

C H A P T E R

6

SPORT-SPECIFIC MASSAGES

Fitness has to be fun. If it is not play, there will be no fitness. Play,
you see, is the process. Fitness is merely the product.

GEORGE SHEEHAN, M.D., *Runner's World*

While more and more people are embracing cross-training—which helps prevent injury as well as staleness—there are still many people who concentrate primarily on one sport. Concentrating on one activity can take its toll on certain areas of the body, as I'm sure you know, and those areas need special attention.

In this chapter I've detailed the specific demands of each sport, explaining what parts of your body need specific attention and why. If you have access to a therapist or a partner who will massage the vulnerable areas, you can have them do the massages listed (refer to chapter 4 for specific directions). Or, if you're on your own, you can use the self-massage routines that I've supplied or use the Thera Cane to massage that body part (see the directions that come with the Thera Cane).

Remember that massage is not a panacea or guarantee against injury. For all sports, you should get into shape gradually and stay in shape with proper stretching and strengthening exercises. Massage should be part of the training process, not a remedy for when things go wrong. Too many sports participants wait until they get injured to turn to massage.

But bear in mind that everything is connected in your body. While you'll want to give these areas special attention or tend to them when you don't have time for a full massage, you'll always benefit from a full-body massage—no matter what your sport.

BICYCLING: FIGHTING OFF STIFFNESS IN ROAD RIDERS

Recommended massage routines: Neck, shoulders, lower back, hands, quadriceps, iliotibial band, hamstrings, buttocks and feet.

Massage has been an integral aspect of training for road and track cycling teams for many years: I was doing massage on a young Greg LeMond back in the 1970s. Part of taking care of yourself as a cyclist is regular massage. Many of the minor aches and pains associated with biking—stiff back, stiff neck, hand numbness—can benefit from massage.

One of my clients, Roch Lockyer, switched from triathlons to concentrate on cycling when he moved to Boulder from Indianapolis. As he increased his miles on the bike, he found that his neck, shoulders and lower back were getting more tight and sore from the specialized training.

The added stress from the cycling position needed to be relieved. I started out by concentrating on Roch's neck, shoulders and lower back. I also helped him visualize relaxing the upper body and talked about the importance of learning to relax both body and mind. Roch learned to relax his upper back while on the bike and let his legs do more of the work, and his style became more effortless. Once the stiffness in his neck, back and shoulders was in check, in later sessions I could move on to concentrate on recovery in the legs.

Because of the road cyclist's bent-over position, the neck is in a constant state of tension to hold the head up. Releasing tension in this area encourages full-body relaxation, facilitating the next training session and improving both recovery and performance.

In cycling, the athlete's body weight is totally supported by the bicycle, so cyclists' muscles will not be as rigid after training as those of runners. But because the body weight is supported, a greater chance of muscle imbalance exists: Often the "stabilizer" muscles will be weak in proportion to the muscles you use to power the bicycle forward.

Road cyclists typically put in exceptionally long training hours (two to three

BICYCLING

NECK—Page 82

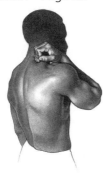

SHOULDERS—Page 83

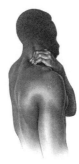

LOWER BACK—Page 80

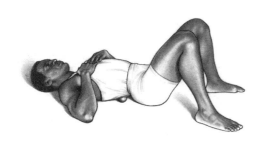

HANDS—Page 76

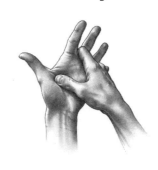

QUADRICEPS—Pages 78, 88

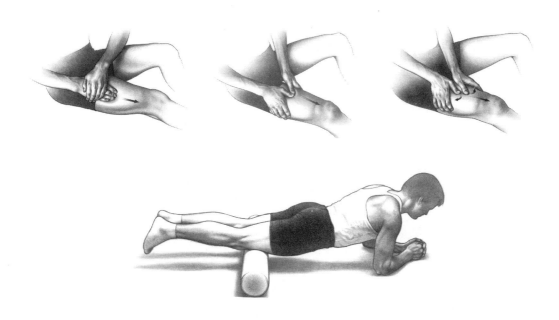

BICYCLING

ILIOTIBIAL BAND—Page 88

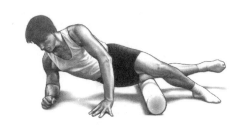

FEET—Page 76

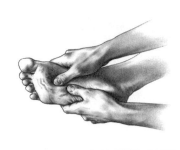

HAMSTRINGS—Pages 79, 86–87

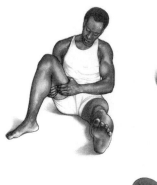

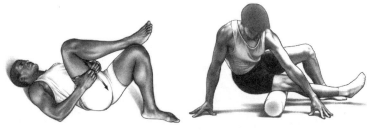

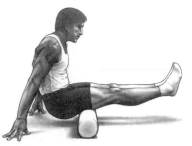

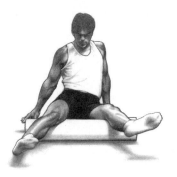

BUTTOCKS—Pages 80, 86

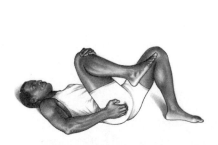

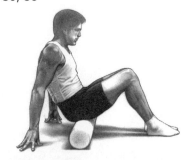

times greater than runners) with a high rpm (100 or more revolutions of the pedals per minute). They require the most work on their legs but may also need particular attention to their feet, as tension may build up from the necessary rigidity of the ankle joint and the tight fit of cycling shoes. Also, hands are often very tender in cyclists, thanks to hours on the handlebars absorbing road vibration and supporting the weight of the upper body.

BODYBUILDING: LIKE KNEADING CONCRETE

Recommended massage routines: All.

The body has 600 muscles, and a bodybuilder uses every one—sometimes three to five days a week, often seven days a week. It's tiring. Also, it pumps up a lot of toxins that massage can flush out. So, no question about it, the bodybuilder needs a full-body massage. But because each workout isolates a particular area, you want to devote proportionately more attention to the muscle group or groups worked on a particular day. (See chapters 4 and 5 for specific routines.)

Incidentally, studies have shown that there are more injuries during pre-exercise stretching than during stretching after exercise. The same rationale applies to post-resistance-training massage: Massage is part of the cooldown.

FIELD AND COURT SPORTS: A WHOLE DIFFERENT BALL GAME

Recommended massage routines: Feet, arms, hands, quadriceps, iliotibial band, hamstrings, buttocks, lower back, neck and chest.

When working on the Colorado College women's soccer team—which was in the Final Four in Division I for seven years—I noted many situations where the players needed increased flexibility. I worked on increasing the range of motion in their hips and their feet via soft-tissue manipulation. This was the first time the coach had suggested massage for his team, and the players began to see that massage was integral to the training process—that by keeping their muscles healthy and flexible, they weren't setting themselves up for injury.

For athletes in field or court sports—which include soccer, lacrosse, field hockey, football, basketball, baseball, tennis, racquetball and squash—the demands on the body are similar to those on runners, but with additional considerations. These sports require endurance, bursts of top-end speed, jumping ability and repeated efforts in a body position with a deeper knee bend than running. The muscular requirements of sprinting require extra attention from the massage thera-pist to encourage recovery or to prepare the muscles for such efforts. Lateral

(continued on page 98)

FIELD AND COURT SPORTS

FEET—Page 76

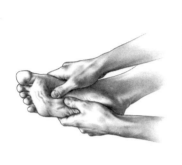

HANDS—Page 76

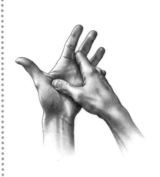

NECK—Page 82

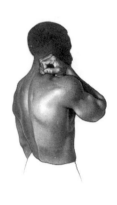

ARMS—Page 81

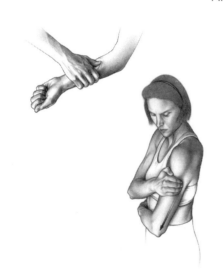

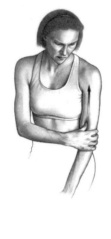

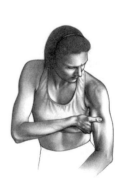

ILIOTIBIAL BAND—Page 88

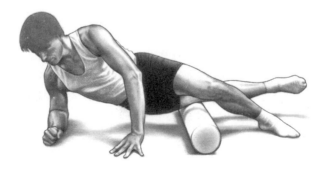

FIELD AND COURT SPORTS

QUADRICEPS—Pages 78, 88

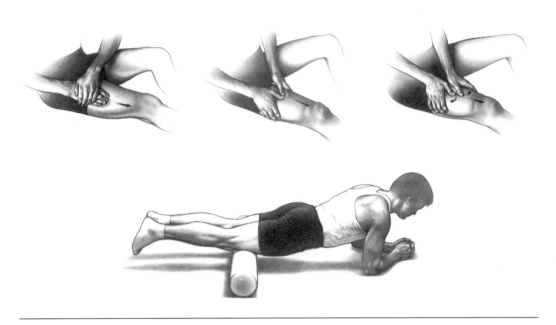

HAMSTRINGS—Pages 79, 86–87

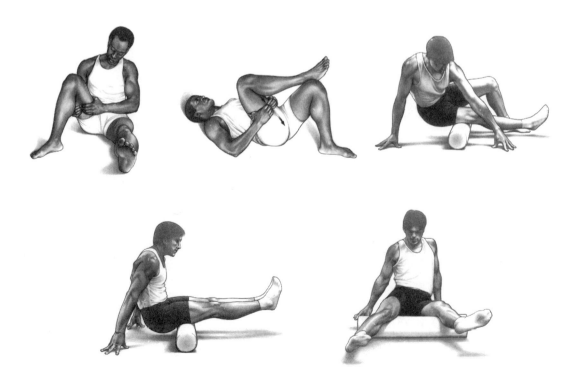

FIELD AND COURT SPORTS

BUTTOCKS—Pages 80, 86

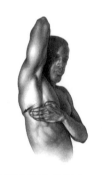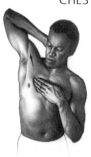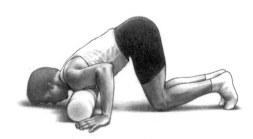

LOWER BACK—Page 80

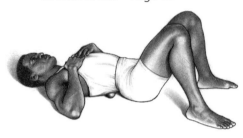

CHEST—Pages 82, 85

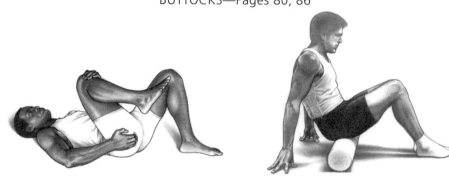

movement and radical direction changes can put stress on the body's stabilizer muscles as well as hip adductors and abductors (which push and pull the hip joint, respectively) and ankle and knee joints. Pounding on a hard surface or the twisting associated with court sports and some field sports warrants extra attention to the feet.

These sports also involve upper-body movement as well as lower-body movement. Athletes in these types of sports should take care not to neglect their upper bodies; they need massage, too.

GOLF: MORE THAN A SWING OF THE HIPS

Recommended massage routines: Hands, forearms, shoulders, feet, buttocks and lower back.

In golf, the power comes from the hips. Yet the gripping action used to grasp golf clubs can do a number on your hands and arms, like the kind of repetitive strain syndrome seen in keyboard operators or other occupations that require a repeated motion. So it's important to treat your hands, forearms and shoulders to regular massage.

Because golf shoes are rigid, like wingtips with spikes, you'll need a foot

GOLF

HANDS—Page 76

FOREARMS—Page 81

SHOULDERS—Page 83

FEET—Page 76

BUTTOCKS—Pages 80, 86

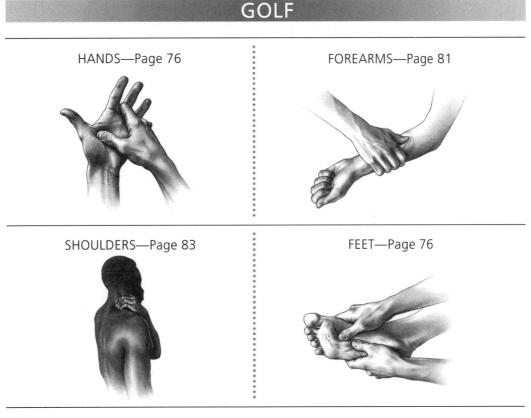
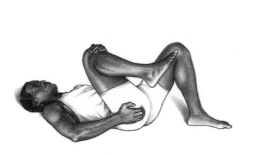
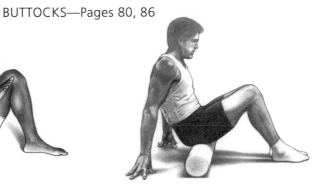

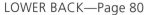

GOLF

LOWER BACK—Page 80

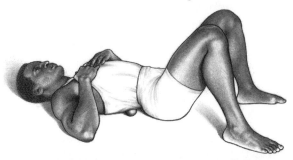

massage after a day of walking the greens. If you carry your clubs in a bag primarily on one side of your body, be sure to massage the side that carries the load (actually, it's a good strategy to switch the bag from one side to the other when you're carrying it). The twisting motion of the golf swing can also take its toll on your lower back. Weekend warriors, especially, have a tendency to strain their backs, so you may want to take special care to do some conditioning and flexibility exercises between games.

GYMNASTICS: FLEXIBILITY IS PARAMOUNT

Recommended massage routines: All.

Gymnastics works both the lower body and the upper body. Male gymnasts, however, tend to concentrate on upper-body routines, with power moves on the horse, rings and parallel bar. When Jesse, an 18-year-old gymnast and Colorado state champion, came to me, he was concerned about a shoulder problem. An orthopedic surgeon he'd consulted recommended surgery for injury to the rotator cuff and deltoid attachments in the shoulder; a physical therapist he'd consulted questioned that recommendation.

When I first started to work with Jesse, he was invariably tight because, as he was going through puberty, gymnastics had shortened his muscles. He had developed collagen, scar tissue and adhesions from enormous amounts of stress and force placed on the body. As a result, he had greatly reduced his natural range of motion. So I spent a lot of extra time on his hands, forearms, upper arms, chest and back—basically freeing up those tight areas. I did a lot of deep-tissue work to try and get the muscle groups to slide past each other with ease instead of being bound together.

Jesse also needed to work on flexibility and incorporating massage with stretching—not so much feet and lower-body massage, but a full-body massage with an extra half-hour on the upper body. As a result, his flexibility increased, and now he's doing great as a freshman gymnast in college.

Female gymnasts, on the other hand, do more floor work—like balance beam routines—that primarily use the lower body, so their massage sessions would concentrate on the legs, feet and lower back. Another benefit of massage for females is that it can improve body image and self-esteem, possibly helping prevent anorexia, which is not uncommon among young women gymnasts.

HIKING AND BACKPACKING: HELP FOR ACHE-ALL-OVER SORENESS

Recommended massage routines: Quadriceps, iliotibial band, feet, back, neck, shoulders and hands.

Alpine hiking—which involves steeper grades than hiking on flat terrain or at lower elevations—mimics running in that it uses many of the same muscle groups, but it's performed more slowly. You have less forceful impact with the surface, but you experience other kinds of strains. Like trail running, hiking takes you uphill and down, using muscle groups that require eccentric contractions, and generally that's what leaves hikers sore. It's going downhill, not uphill, that hurts. Specifically, the quads and knees may hurt, especially the iliotibial band, which stretches from just below the knee to the hip and runs along the outside of the thigh.

Downhill hiking can aggravate chondromalacia patellae (a softening of the cartilage covering the underside of the kneecap, commonly known as runner's knee) or patellar tendinitis (inflammation of the tendon that connects the lower and upper patellar tendons in the kneecap to the femur, or thigh bone). If you have either of these problems, you'll want to check with a sports podiatrist or sports medicine specialist.

Hiking boots lend ankle support (which is good), but heavier boots can add weight and therefore stress to the knee joint (not so good). Obviously, both ankles and knees will benefit from massage, no matter what type of boot you use. For iliotibial band soreness, self-massage—especially with ice—is just the ticket.

If you carry a pack of any kind—and even day hikers should carry water, basic first aid and extra outer gear for unexpected delays or weather changes— you'll want a back and neck massage. The heavier the pack, the greater the strain on the shoulders and entire back. When you get home from your hike, you can use an Ethafoam roller to massage your back (see the illustrations on pages 102 and 103, or

HIKING AND BACKPACKING

QUADRICEPS—Pages 78, 88

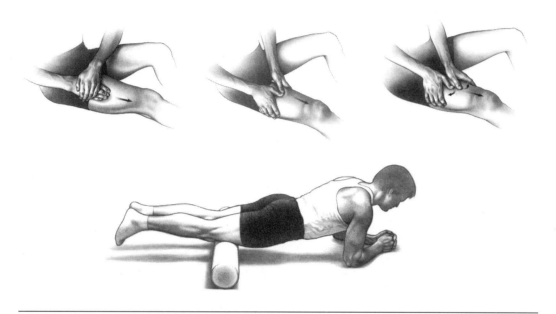

ILIOTIBIAL BAND—Page 88

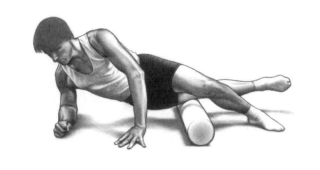

FEET—Page 76

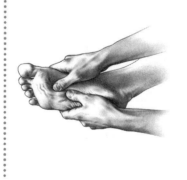

UPPER BACK—Page 84

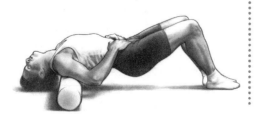

MIDDLE BACK—Page 85

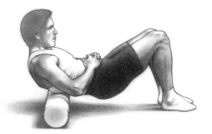

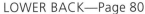

HIKING AND BACKPACKING

LOWER BACK—Page 80

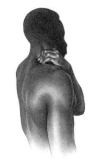

NECK—Page 82

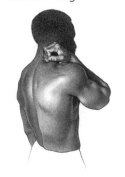

SHOULDERS—Page 83

HANDS—Page 76

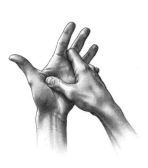

refer to chapter 5). Another good trick is to hold a racquetball against the wall with your back and roll it around by bending and straightening your legs; you could even carry a ball in your pack and use a handy tree!

Whether you backpack or take day hikes, a foot massage will relieve some of the stress from the day's work. Finally, if you use a hiking staff, ski pole or poles or carry a camera, your hands and arms may also need attention.

KAYAKING AND ROWING: TLC FOR THE WRISTS

Recommended massage routines: Hands, forearms, shoulders, back, neck and chest.

The entire upper body from the hips up provides the power for kayaking and rowing. You use the hips a considerable amount to direct and steady the boat, and paddlers can experience overuse injuries of the tendons in the hands, wrists, shoulders and forearms.

More often than not, safety dictates that you'll be out with a friend (especially for ocean kayaking), so if you're on an overnight trip you can get your

KAYAKING AND ROWING

HANDS—Page 76

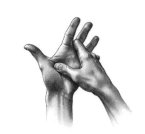

FOREARMS—Page 81

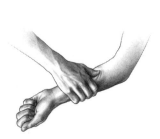

SHOULDERS—Page 83

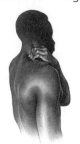

UPPER BACK—Page 84

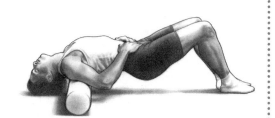

MIDDLE BACK—Page 85

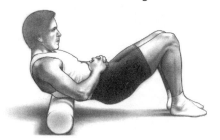

LOWER BACK—Page 80

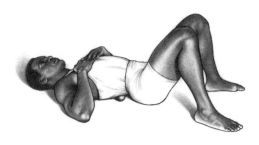

NECK—Page 82

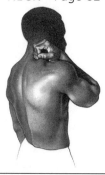

CHEST—Pages 82,85

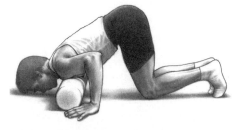
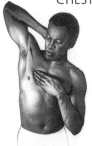

paddling partner to help with massage techniques. For shorter trips, of course, you can get someone to massage you as soon as you get home. Otherwise, you can turn to self-massage.

Sports such as kayaking that use primarily the upper body may also stress the ankles, knees, legs, hips and spine. Treating the entire body to the occasional massage, as with all sports, will encourage recovery of the muscular system as a whole.

MOUNTAIN BIKING: THE SHAKING TAKES A TOLL

Recommended massage routines: Hands, forearms, quadriceps, iliotibial band, hamstrings, lower back, buttocks, neck and shoulders.

Mountain bikers, especially racers and hard-core riders, have specific needs. I attended the 1994 World Mountain Biking Championships at Vail, Colorado, and I'd never seen the kind of rattling and shaking I witnessed at those races—the whole body vibrates. Of course, most recreational mountain bikers won't experience the degree of trauma that serious competitors do, but after a day on the trails you will feel the effects—especially if you work hard to clear obstacles, climb, descend and corner with panache instead of walking the bike.

Mountain bikers experience many of the same lower-body strains as road cyclists do—they're just going more slowly and using their bodies to push and pull the bike more. The most common complaints among mountain bikers are soreness in the hands, wrists and forearms, plus some shoulder stiffness. Also, the iliotibial band gets very irritated or inflamed because, like skaters, mountain bikers make heavy use of the hip adductor muscles to pull the legs in. Carl Yarbrough, a sports photographer and accomplished mountain biker, came to me for work on his iliotibial band, and it helped him considerably.

MOUNTAIN BIKING

HANDS—Page 76

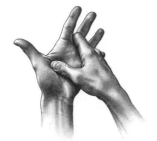

FOREARMS—Page 81

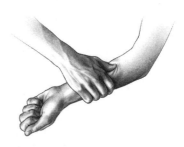

MOUNTAIN BIKING

QUADRICEPS—Pages 78, 88

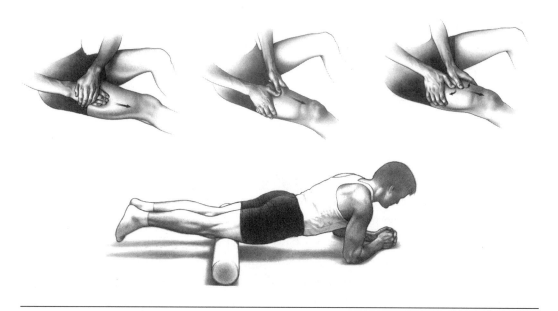

HAMSTRINGS—Pages 79, 86–87

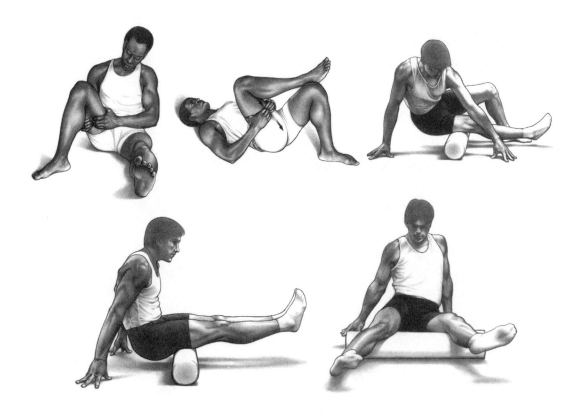

MOUNTAIN BIKING

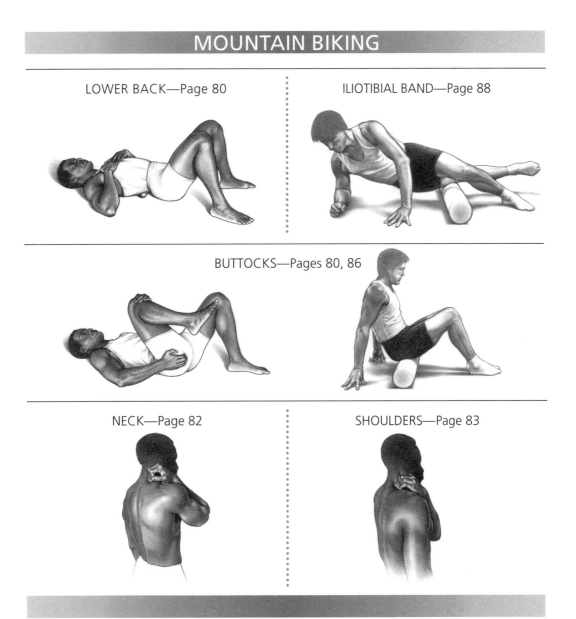

LOWER BACK—Page 80

ILIOTIBIAL BAND—Page 88

BUTTOCKS—Pages 80, 86

NECK—Page 82

SHOULDERS—Page 83

ROCK AND MOUNTAIN CLIMBING: TREATING "CLIMBER'S WRIST"

Recommended massage routines: Arms, hands, chest, neck, shoulders, upper back, lower back and feet.

When top-ranked climber Robyn Erbesfield came to me, she had some tennis elbow–like symptoms that were restricting her hand and wrist motion. I used a variety of techniques in her massage treatment, and Robyn was able to compete with ease in a sport-climbing competition the following weekend in Berkeley, California—and win handily.

ROCK AND MOUNTAIN CLIMBING

ARMS—Page 81

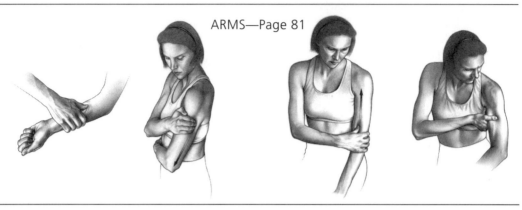

CHEST—Pages 82, 85

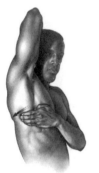
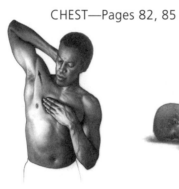
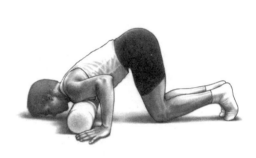

HANDS—Page 76

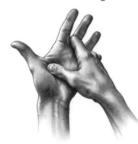

FEET—Page 76

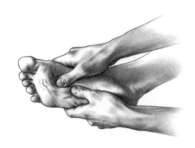

NECK—Page 82

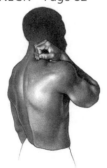

SHOULDERS—Page 83

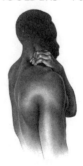

ROCK AND MOUNTAIN CLIMBING

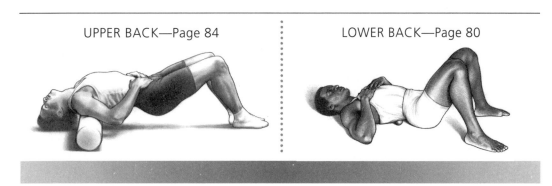

UPPER BACK—Page 84

LOWER BACK—Page 80

her forearm muscles. Once I started palpating those muscles, I could tell by feel exactly what needed to be worked on. Developing this sense of touch takes time and patience, but it's well worth it.

In rock climbing, exceptional stress is exerted on the muscles of the upper body from almost constant use of the arms, shoulders and hands. You need to constantly consider and treat these areas to prevent overuse injuries.

Massage will encourage recovery of the arms and shoulders, and should help prevent future injuries caused by overuse. Tension in these areas will undoubtedly hamper the performance of rock climbers and hinder them in recovering from hard efforts.

RUNNING: CONCENTRATE ON THE LEGS

Recommended massage routines: Feet, calves, shins, quadriceps, iliotibial band, hamstrings, buttocks, lower back.

At the Boulder Bolder 10-K in 1993, Frank Shorter hobbled up to me, holding his calf muscle. He had just finished the race, really whaling it during the last part. "My calf has really tightened up on me," he said, explaining that, as founder of the race, it was especially important that he hadn't given up. "Would you have time to check this out?" he asked.

When Frank showed up for his appointment, I asked him if he had received much massage. "No," he replied, "but if I were to do things differently, I probably would make more time for massage."

For the moment, Frank's goal was immediate relief. He explained that his calf had been bothering him for about six months, and after I did a full-body massage, it became apparent that both his sciatic nerves were severely impinged. Apparently, his calves weren't getting their full blood supply, and the muscles had started to atrophy.

For the next ten weeks I worked on Frank once a week, and it took me those ten weeks to "normalize" the tissue and muscle balance. What's normal, and how do you know you've reached it? It's like baking bread: The baker knows by feel when the bread dough is ready to throw in the oven. Now Frank comes regularly for his dose of "preventive maintenance."

When running first became popular, many people developed running injuries. Lacking proper training information, people made many mistakes. In particular, enthusiasts tended to run longer, harder and more often than their bodies could tolerate.

But running itself doesn't cause injuries. Through a sensibly progressive training program, the body can adapt to extremes. But when the stress becomes too great or is introduced too rapidly, the body will try to escape the stress-creating activity through mechanical breakdown. Injuries are predictable under such circumstances.

Traumatized by repeated stress, shock and vibration, connective tissues may become inflamed and muscles may remain in a semicontracted state, even after training is completed. When this tension-holding pattern becomes the body's norm, your performance and tolerance will become permanently limited. The muscular tension associated with running requires that the therapist work the entire body: upper back, lower back, buttocks, hamstrings, calves, shins and feet. Massage encourages the muscles to relax, thereby helping the athlete recover from the last training session and prepare for the next one.

The top of the shin is often tender in runners. Loosening this spot alleviates much of the tension and discomfort on the shin and relieves or prevents pain in this area, often called shinsplints.

If you've already developed a running injury, you'll want to visit a physical therapist or sports medicine doctor, of course. I also recommend *Running Injury-Free* by Joe Ellis and Joe Henderson.

RUNNING

FEET—Page 76

CALVES—Page 77

RUNNING

SHINS—Page 77

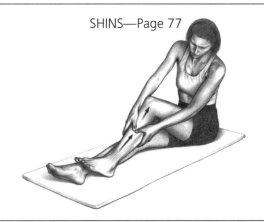

QUADRICEPS—Pages 78, 88

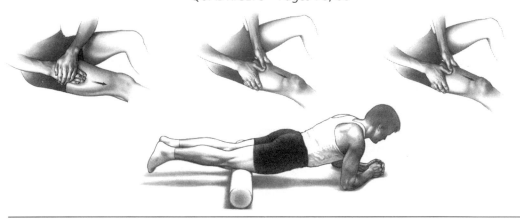

HAMSTRINGS—Pages 79, 86–87

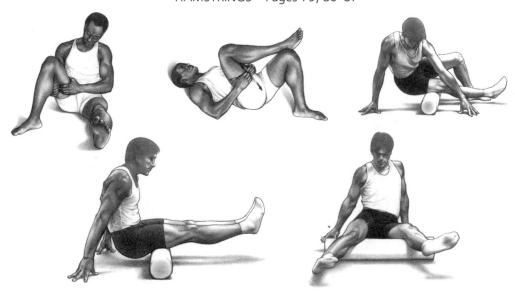

RUNNING

ILIOTIBIAL BAND—Page 88

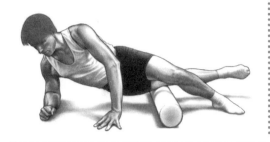

LOWER BACK—Page 80

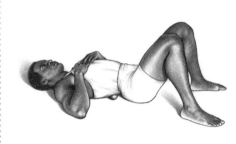

BUTTOCKS—Pages 80, 86

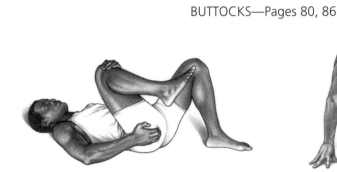

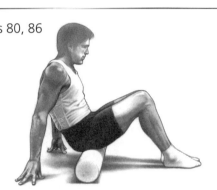

SKATING: FOOT, LEG AND BACK MAINTENANCE

Recommended massage routines: Lower back, buttocks, hamstrings, quadriceps, calves, iliotibial band, inner thighs, shins, feet, ankles, neck and shoulders.

In nearly every athlete, the lower back is not as strong as it should be. Nowhere is this more apparent than in skaters, whether figure, hockey, speed or in-line skater. The buttocks and hamstrings are the primary muscles involved in propulsion in any skating technique. This plus the skater's tendency to bend forward to accommodate the laterally oriented skating stroke puts tremendous stresses on the lower back.

The muscle activity associated with long, gliding strokes puts great stress on the quadriceps, while the sideways nature of the skating stroke tests the hip flexors, iliotibial band and muscles involved in abduction and adduction. Maintaining these areas through massage helps the skater avoid knee problems that may be associated with quadriceps and iliotibial band tightening.

Skaters' feet suffer from being cramped into tight skates. Skates are typically laced tighter than normal footwear to ensure ankle support, so some special attention to both feet and ankles is warranted (see pages 49 and 50 for ankle massages). Figure skater Jill Trenary was a client of mine for four years, and her goal was to make the Olympic team as well as win a world championship. She was referred to me by a physical therapist, who thought that over the long run Jill might be able to train harder with the benefits of massage. Jill had some scar tissue buildup in the ankle area, specifically from the tight lacing of skates. The first order of business was to address Jill's tight foot muscles and scar tissue. From there I went on to general massage to facilitate recovery.

Over the course of the first year Jill came to me for massage therapy, she experienced far fewer injuries than the previous season, and she credits this partially to the powers of massage. Jill later went on to win the 1991 World Championships and has placed fourth twice in the Olympics.

Tightly laced skates can also affect the calves and shins, though many calf and shin problems are more closely related to stress generated in maintaining balance. Massage encourages relaxation in these areas, and it could prevent injuries from occurring.

Because of the bent-forward position used by skaters, the neck is forced to remain tense in elevating the head through the duration of training. Releasing tension in this area encourages full-body relaxation, facilitating the next training session and improving both recovery and performance.

SKATING

LOWER BACK—Page 80

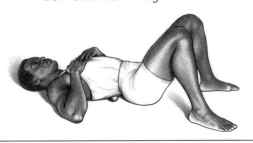

BUTTOCKS—Pages 80, 86

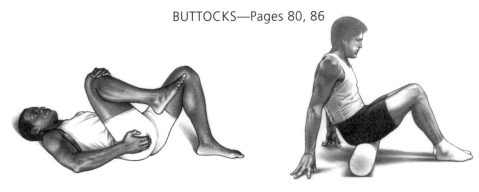

SKATING

HAMSTRINGS—Pages 79, 86–87

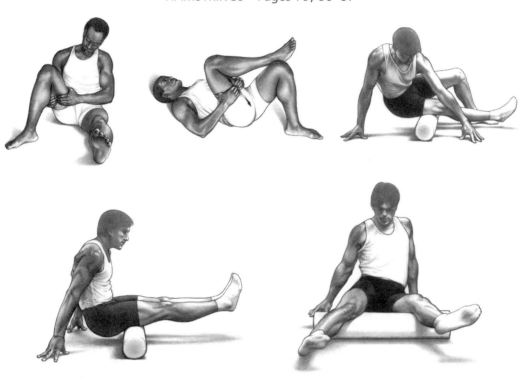

QUADRICEPS—Pages 78, 88

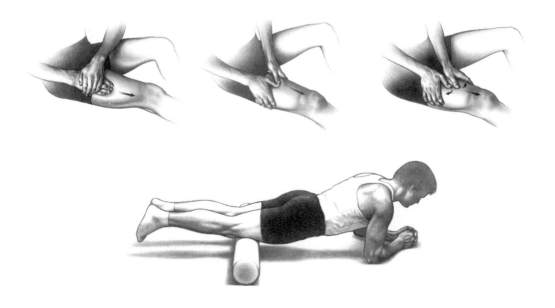

SKATING

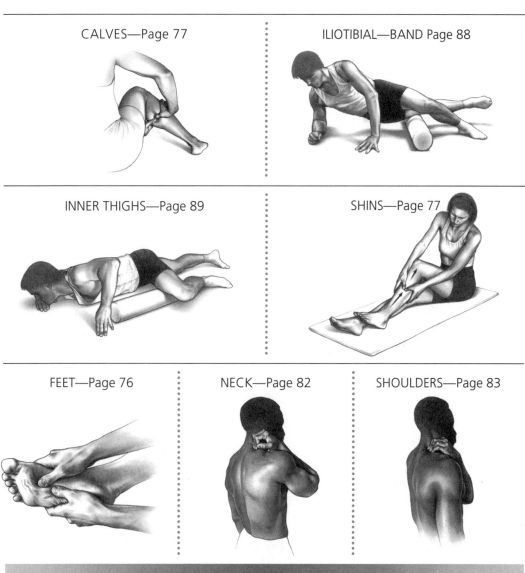

CALVES—Page 77

ILIOTIBIAL—BAND Page 88

INNER THIGHS—Page 89

SHINS—Page 77

FEET—Page 76

NECK—Page 82

SHOULDERS—Page 83

SKIING (CROSS-COUNTRY): THE WHOLE-BODY WORKOUT

Recommended massage routines: All.

I met four-time Olympian Lyle Nelson at a summer biathlon competition; this was my first exposure to a winter biathlete, whose sport involves skiing and shooting. I thought I knew skiing, but I had to visualize the impact of carrying an object that you use with one side of your body—the rifle—like a tennis player who is dominant on one side. In certain sports muscle imbalances occur, and I noticed that Lyle's right arm and lats (latissimus dorsi) were overdeveloped, much like a tennis player's.

One of the things that I realized from working with Lyle was the amazing amount of muscle mass that is used in skiing, one of the most demanding sports when it comes to VO_2 max, the capacity of the lungs and circulatory system to take in oxygen and deliver it to the muscles for use.

Cross-country skiing has been described as the perfect whole-body sport: It works just about every muscle in your body. So for this sport, you're generally going to need a full-body massage rather than concentrating on one part of the body. However, you may have one area that's particularly sore, depending on your own fitness level. Your legs, for instance, may be hardy from hours of road cycling, but the relatively unused muscles in your arms may scream from the unaccustomed demands of poling after your first day out skiing this winter.

SKIING (DOWNHILL): HELP FOR SCREAMING QUADS

Recommended massage routines: Quadriceps, iliotibial band, calves, shins, buttocks, hamstrings, back, feet, neck and shoulders.

In alpine skiing particularly, athletes can suffer cramped and tense feet from the restrictive nature of ski boots. Calves and shins may require extra attention after long days of tensing to maintain balance. Knees are often sore and swollen, requiring extra attention to the quadriceps and iliotibial bands. Even if your knees can take the pounding, your quads may scream in agony, especially when you try to walk down stairs or inclines. The lower back and buttocks may be tense and sore from the pounding and static muscle activity of alpine skiing.

In fact, the most common complaint I get from downhill skiers is about pain in their backs: They tell me that after a day on the slopes, they feel as if they've been doing construction work all day.

Tension associated with maintaining balance often accumulates in the neck and shoulders. Massaging this area frequently enhances both recovery and performance. Work on the legs, of course, will make up the majority of any skier's massage, but you may also have to work on exhausted upper arms, forearms and hands.

Muscle soreness among skiers is often a result of pushing too hard too soon. Many skiers are tempted to spend as much time as possible on the slopes or the trail, with few breaks. Gentle massage can be beneficial in treating knots and stiff spots as well as the soreness from the repeated spills and crashes that many of us associate with skiing.

DOWNHILL SKIING

QUADRICEPS—Pages 78, 88

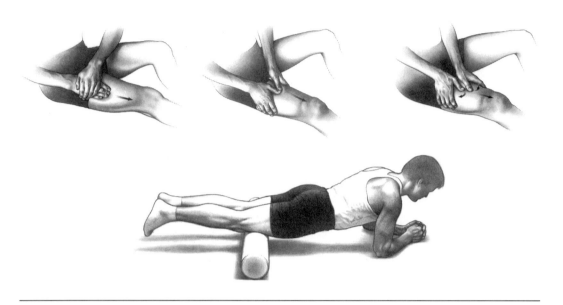

ILIOTIBIAL BAND—Page 88

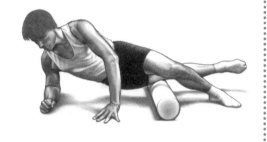

CALVES—Page 77

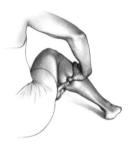

SHINS—Page 77

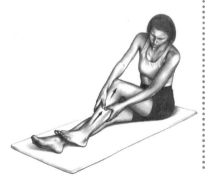

BUTTOCKS—Pages 80,86

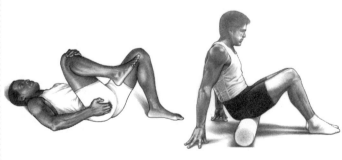

DOWNHILL SKIING

HAMSTRINGS—Pages 79, 86–87

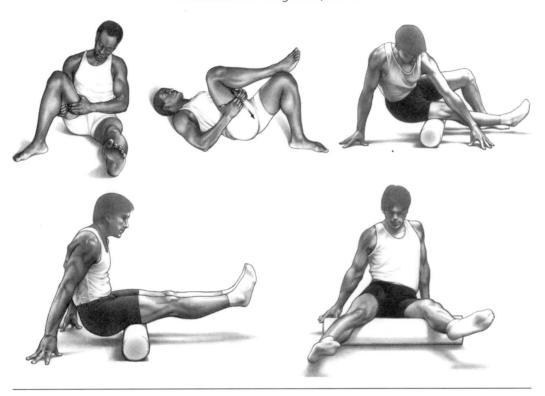

UPPER BACK—Page 84

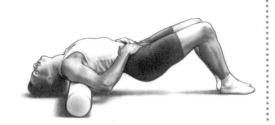

MIDDLE BACK—Page 85

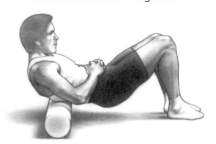

LOWER BACK—Page 80

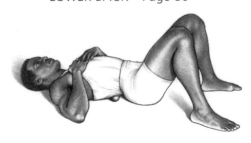

DOWNHILL SKIING

FEET—Page 76

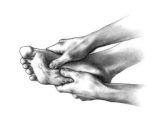

NECK—Page 82

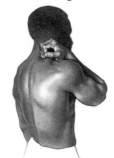

SHOULDERS—Page 83

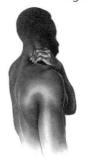

SWIMMING: RELIEF FOR SHOULDER WOES

Recommended massage routines: Shoulders, arms, neck, back, buttocks, feet and hands.

Eric Hansen was helping conduct studies for the swimming flume at the U.S. Olympic Center in Colorado Springs when I met him. Eric, who later went on to receive a Ph.D. in sports medicine, wanted to qualify for not only the U.S. swimming trials but also the U.S. team slated to attend the 1992 Barcelona Olympics. Eric used massage religiously to help him recover so that each hard workout would advance him further toward that goal.

Eric originally came to me complaining of stiffness in the rotator cuff and general soreness in the shoulders. Massage took care of those relatively minor problems and helped him recover more quickly for the next workout. As it turned out, Eric didn't make the team, but he felt good about the effort he was able to put forth, unimpeded by injury.

In swimming, the athlete's weight is supported by the water's natural buoyancy, so there is no pounding to contend with. There is, however, the accumulated strain of tremendous repetition. Most of the strain experienced by swimmers is in the upper body.

Degradation of the shoulder joint and injuries to muscles of the shoulder girdle and upper arm are not uncommon among swimmers. In no way should injuries such as these be addressed by a massage therapist until the client has been examined by a physician. Consistent massage of the shoulder, back and arm muscles, however, may help prevent injuries from occurring. Massage helps alleviate pressure inside the joint by relaxing the muscles associated with that joint.

Much of each stroke's propulsion is derived from the arms. Following a workout, swimmers generally are exhausted in the arms, chest and shoulders. Massage encourages recovery of these muscle systems. Hands and feet may be prone to cramping from the effects of pushing against the water. Also, there may be some stiffness in the buttocks and lower back, as the kicking stroke in swimming is generated primarily by the muscles originating in the pelvic girdle and lower back.

SWIMMING

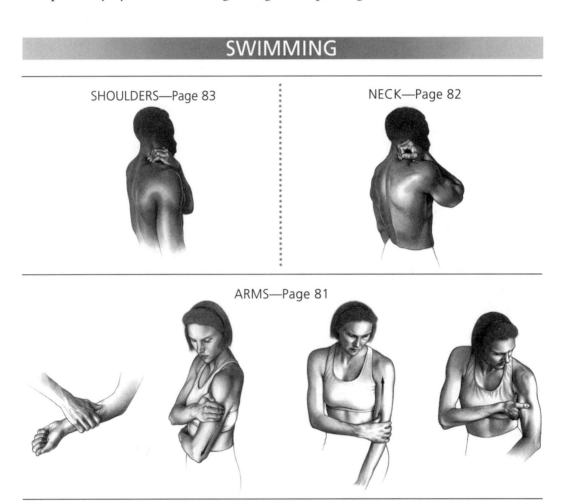

SHOULDERS—Page 83

NECK—Page 82

ARMS—Page 81

UPPER BACK—Page 84

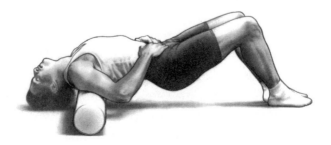

SWIMMING

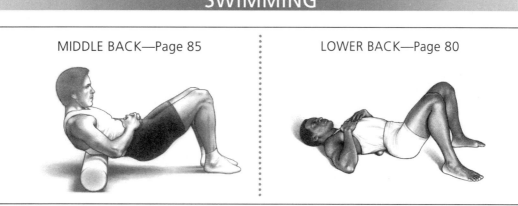

MIDDLE BACK—Page 85

LOWER BACK—Page 80

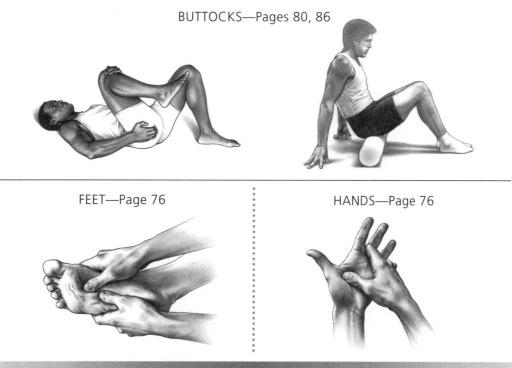

BUTTOCKS—Pages 80, 86

FEET—Page 76

HANDS—Page 76

VOLLEYBALL: WHOLE-BODY POWER MOVES

Recommended massage routines: Shoulders, back, calves, quadriceps, buttocks and feet.

In volleyball, every part of the body comes into play. The upper body, especially the shoulders and back, provides a great deal of power. Rotator cuff injuries are a big problem. But the biggest complaint is back problems from the explosive plyometric-type movement required—leaping and bounding, in everyday terms. In that respect, volleyball is like football or other sprint sports. But the calves provide as much power as the upper body because players are constantly on their toes.

Many volleyball players experience overuse injuries in the wrists. Plus, in court volleyball, players wear very snugly fitting shoes on a hard wooden floor, so their feet take a pounding. In beach volleyball, sand is a therapeutic medium—it provides a sort of massage for the feet during play.

VOLLEYBALL

SHOULDERS—Page 83

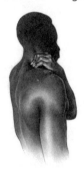

UPPER BACK—Page 84

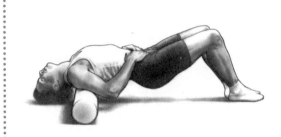

MIDDLE BACK—Page 85

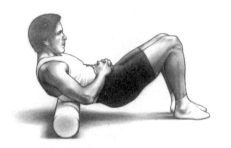

LOWER BACK—Page 80

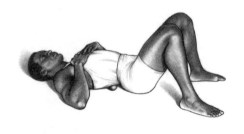

CALVES—Page 77

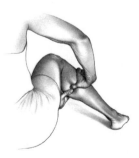

FEET Page—76

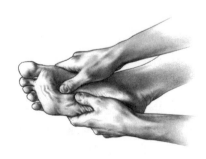

VOLLEYBALL

QUADRICEPS—Pages 78, 88

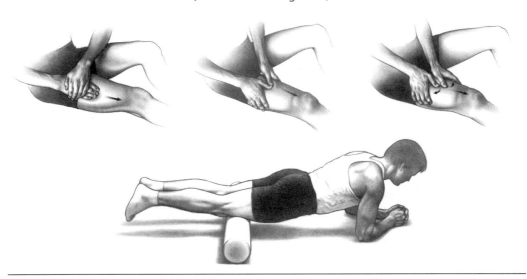

BUTTOCKS—Pages 80, 86

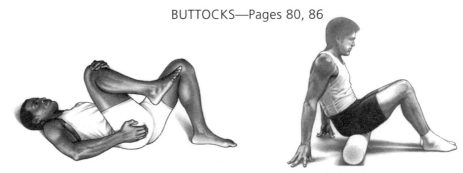

WINDSURFING: HELP FOR THE HUMAN SAILBOAT

Recommended massage routines: Calves, buttocks, quadriceps, feet, neck and shoulders, back, arms and hands.

As with cyclists, windsurfers stabilize themselves with their legs. They also give their feet a workout, so massage of the entire lower body is useful.

To keep the board upright, windsurfers make extra use of their forearms, like rock climbers. And both the biceps and triceps (antagonistic muscles) are engaged, along with the deltoids, while the neck and lower back are hyperextended. Windsurfers can also be subject to repetitive strain injuries to their forearms, although use of a harness can help take some of the strain off their arms.

WINDSURFING

BUTTOCKS—Pages 80, 86

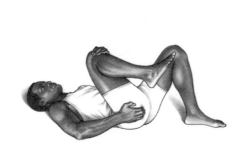
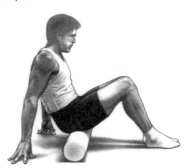

CALVES—Page 77

FEET—Page 76

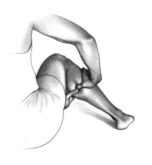
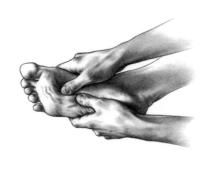

QUADRICEPS—Pages 78, 88

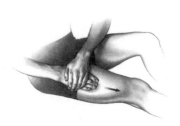
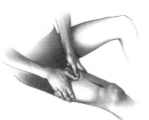
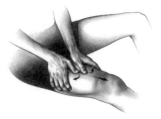

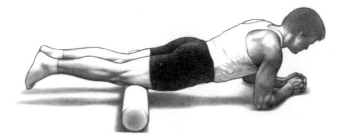

WINDSURFING

NECK—Page 82

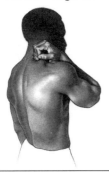

SHOULDERS—Page 83

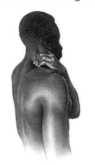

HANDS—Page 76

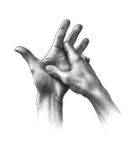

UPPER BACK—Page 84

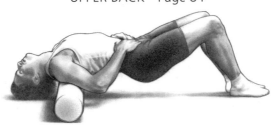

MIDDLE BACK—Page 85

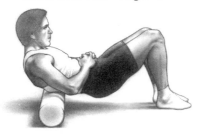

LOWER BACK—Page 80

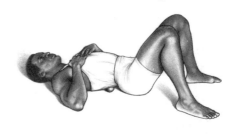

ARMS—Page 81

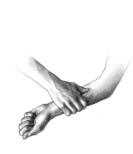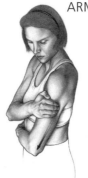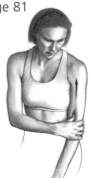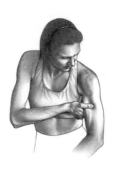

7

RECOVERY FROM HARD EFFORTS

Exercise is work, but it is also pleasure, and pleasure is the part that keeps us at it.

JOHN JEROME, *Staying Supple*

Everyone, from the weekend warrior to the world-record holder, is going to overdo it eventually. Pushing yourself to the max—or beyond—may be deliberate or it may be accidental, but once you have overdone it—at work, at play or during training—you'll know it.

If you simply come home from working out and lie down on the couch, you'll eventually recover from overextending yourself. But for most athletes, simple rest and recovery aren't good enough. Recovering more quickly allows you to get back to serious training as soon as possible. The sooner you recover from the last hard effort, the sooner you can get on to the next. And if recovering quickly is your goal, then something a bit more methodical and ambitious than "couch rehab" is required.

Symptoms of hard effort include muscle soreness, mild spasm, fatigue, stiffness, limited range of motion and a general lethargy. The quicker you overcome these obstacles, the better. The four most widely accepted practices to speed recovery from hard efforts are rest, ice, compression and elevation (commonly referred to as RICE). Sports massage can assist and contribute to these four methods, especially when used in tandem with another wonderful recovery tool, hydrotherapy.

MASSAGE AND REST: A TIME TO RECOVER

The body responds to the stresses of hard efforts by developing higher levels of ability and tolerance, which generally translates into improved overall performance. For maximum gains in performance, however, you must allow your muscles enough time to recover.

Top distance runner Arturo Barrios lists rest as one of the key factors in his equation for success. The other ingredients are proper diet, training, massage and mental preparation. "Regular rest is the main factor in recovery," he says. "I like to take three to four weeks completely off at the end of the year to regenerate and rebuild depleted reserves." Your own recipe for rest and recovery might mean running slowly once a day, he points out, or seeking out other forms of exercise and ways to keep active, such as basketball, cycling or swimming. Besides his annual month-long break from running, Arturo regularly swims, visits the steam room and whirlpool, and of course has his twice-weekly massages.

When you're training, the body is in the catabolic state; that is, cells convert substances into simpler ones and release energy. Following training, during the anabolic, or growth, state, the body is more inclined toward repair than toward further training. During rest, muscles are repaired and return to normal lengths, and joints return to normal ranges of motion. If you refuse to spend sufficient time in the resting, anabolic state following hard efforts, the body will reach a point where it will resist further gains and training will produce only fatigue. In plain English, you'll burn out.

After extraordinary efforts, you're going to need passive rest, during which your body will be drawing on every available resource to heal itself. Passive rest means resting and nothing else. Active rest, a period of light activity designed to allow the muscles to recover, should be a part of every week's training program between training sessions of higher intensity.

What role does massage play in the rest phase? Massage is generally recommended as a recovery tool one to three hours after intense exercise. That gives you time to warm down completely and spend some quiet recovery time in passive rest before the massage. A period of passive rest will signal the body and its systems that the work has been completed and that repair and recovery can begin. After this, massage will be most effective.

MASSAGE WITH ICE: PUT OUT THE FIRE

Heat is a natural bodily reaction to injuries and stresses. Discomfort is the body's way of telling you that you went too far and you need to recover. Your body is smart in wanting to recover from the last bout of work before going on to the next one.

Inflammation is signal numero uno among the body's various whines and creaks; swelling results from the tendency of each cell, under stress, to soak up as much intracellular fluid as it can accommodate, stretching the cell walls and causing the cell to bump vigorously into neighboring cells. Just like a room occupied by too many people, the stressed area begins to overheat. The temperature rises locally and circulation increases to the inflamed area.

Ice cools the inflamed area and decreases local circulation, thereby relieving the discomfort. After ice is removed from the inflamed area, normal circulation resumes, allowing the blood to cleanse the area of waste products, such as lactic acid. Lactic acid dissipates within 30 minutes after a hard effort. (Some feel it actually serves as a kind of "fuel" for further effort.) But plenty of toxins produced by hard effort remain; they need to be carried away before recovery can begin.

Each session of intense exercise produces some damage. Minute tears occur in the muscles, joints swell slightly and mobility is decreased. This is normal. And repair of these damaged tissues is an integral part of athletic improvement. Your body isn't stupid—it's like the people whose houses are flattened by an earthquake. When they rebuild them, they make them stronger, able to withstand the next quake. Fortunately for you, your body has the ability to withstand nearly countless numbers of "earthquakes," given the proper amount of time for rebuilding.

Ice massage is one of the safest, cheapest, fastest and most readily available means of preventing swelling, reducing pain and decreasing the intensity of muscle soreness associated with overuse. It has become a widely accepted and sometimes superior alternative to traditional ice therapy (where ice is merely applied to the area) and can be used in any situation that might normally suggest application of ice packs. Ice massage has also been shown to do a better job of transmitting the cold to your tissues than ice packs, thus increasing the therapeutic effects. And, of course, it's a form of self-massage.

To perform ice massage: Keep water frozen in Styrofoam or paper cups in your freezer. Massage the target area with the ice on the open end of the cup in a circular motion until the area begins to feel numb. Tear away the top rim of the cup as the ice melts down. The length of an ice massage varies with the individual and depends upon the area of the body being treated. Typical duration of a single treatment is 10 to 20 minutes. One 10-minute application may be enough, or you may want to continue the ice massage in a pattern of 15 minutes on, 15 minutes off, for one hour. If you ice a muscle (one that is not seriously injured), be sure to gently stretch it afterward.

To help prevent injuries, use ice massage to treat the areas that have been stressed during exercise or that are prone to stiffness, soreness or injury. By cooling areas of minor damage and then increasing circulation to flush out the "gunk," you decrease the low-level swelling that occurs after all intense exercise and lessen the chances of problems or injuries occurring in the future. Use ice massage as soon as possible after warm-down. The goal is to treat the swelling that is bound to occur following intense exercise before the body has time to beat you to the punch. Swelling is easier to prevent than it is to get rid of.

A precaution: Prolonged contact of ice with the skin after numbness has occurred can result in frostbite. Furthermore, skin that has suffered frostbite in the past will be more sensitive to temperature extremes. While ice massage can be an important element in recovery from hard efforts, take care not to "burn" your skin. To be safe, don't exceed more than 15 to 20 minutes of constant ice massage. Generally, however, most athletes will grow bored with ice massage long before they've done too much.

MASSAGE AS COMPRESSION: SQUEEZE THE SPONGE

Under stress, muscle cells absorb intracellular fluids like little sponges, gorging themselves with as much as they can hold as a buffer against damage. In time, muscles eventually recover—inflammation subsides, and accumulated toxins and waste products generated by exercise are flushed out. But you can speed up the process. The most straightforward way to accomplish this is to squeeze the "sponge." This is where compression comes in.

Standard methods of compression include use of support hose, bandage wraps or direct manual pressure. Part of the reason that ice massage is so popular is that it, too, compresses the area. But massage itself serves as a means of compression. Massage restricts local blood flow, flushes waste products from tissues, and temporarily interrupts involuntary electronic impulses that create tiny spasms causing "knots." So massage is often recommended for mild soreness, prevention of potential injury and treatment for diagnosed injury.

It's crucial to communicate closely with the person you're massaging so that your efforts will produce the most benefit for the athlete's recovery. If you're not sure about how vigorously they want to be massaged, err on the side of gentleness.

Massage and Elevation: Make Gravity Work for You

Athletes in nearly every sport spend a maddening amount of effort working against gravity—lifting, climbing, throwing and vaulting. Elevation is a way to harness this typically annoying physical force for good effect. By elevating the complaining body parts—tired legs, swollen feet, a tennis elbow—after intense exercise, gravity will act to reverse the flow of blood and counter the physiological responses to intense exercise. To get gravity working against the flow of blood, it's best to position the affected area higher than the heart. Simply put, sitting on the couch with your feet up is better than hanging your feet over the edge, but lying on the floor with your feet up on the couch is better still.

Elevation is recommended for any body part, after any exercise and as soon after exercise as possible following a full warm-down. There is no limit to the amount of time that elevation is beneficial. The simplest guideline is that elevation is always useful following exercise, either as a measure to prevent overuse injuries in the future or as an active part of recovery. When the dogs are barking, put 'em up.

The Healing Benefits of Water Massage

The goal of this book is to make wellness and self-healing available and understandable for as many people as possible. In that vein, it is important to point out the therapeutic tool that is available to almost everyone—water. Where water is concerned, the advice that "if it feels good, do it" is not only apropros, it's welcome.

The guidelines are pretty simple: Use cold water for pain or injury and hot water for muscle relaxation. Hydrotherapy (as water therapy is aptly referred to) can mean a hot shower, cold shower, sauna, hot tub or steam bath. Soak your feet or hands or head. Stand in a creek and let the current freeze and massage those sore ankles, knees and shins. Take a swim in the local pool, walk in the shallow end, run in the deep end—your body craves the presence and properties of water, internally and externally, and its presence is certainly therapeutic. The movement of water on the body has many of the same healing properties as a light massage. And water moving over the surface of the body is like a tonic, both mentally and physically. I like to think of the flow of the water as a gentle, soothing massage.

Kim Jones, top American female finisher at the Boston, London and Chicago Marathons, uses water as a sort of all-over ice massage. "I'll stick the lower half of my body into the river and get it all done at once," she says. The cool temperature and the massagelike qualities of moving water combine to make this an excellent post-workout therapy.

· ·

KEEP YOUR TANK FILLED UP

All the rest and ice and compression (massage) and elevation in the world won't do much good unless you conscientiously replace the elements that have been depleted during exercise.

In determining how, when and with what to replenish, you will find as many opinions as you find people to ask. There is no secret formula, nor any magic elixir. Perhaps the best advice is to listen to your body, be knowledgeable about the particular demands of exercise on your body, respond to logical cravings (a craving for pasta, a hunger for red meat, a sudden yen for sweets) and be sensible about rehydration and nutrition.

Massage makes your muscles more receptive to restoration at the cellular level. Therefore, it is important to replenish fluids after massage, just as it is important to replenish them after exercise. The fluids in your body will be carrying waste products and toxins that are released from muscle tissues by massage. Increasing your water intake will lower this toxicity and lessen the strain on your filtering organs. Recovery from hard exercise is a chemical process, and every bodily chemical process is facilitated by the presence of water. As a tool in recovery, hydration is indispensable.

The actual recovery of the muscles is a process of repair of damaged tissue. To repair broken-down muscle fiber requires that you eat the right foods. Aerobic exercise will deplete glycogen stores, so replenish after aerobic exercise with carbohydrate sources. But remember that muscle damage occurs during intense exercise and that the fuel required in muscle repair is protein. Be sure to make room in your diet for the protein that is so vital for muscle repair. Most dietitians recommend a diet of 20 percent protein, 30 percent fat and 50 percent carbohydrates for the general public, although sports nutritionists will urge less fat and more carbohydrates.

· ·

Many athletes, particularly those in sports where injuries are often impact-related, have begun using hydrotherapy as a gentle element of both cross-training and recovery. Water workouts, including swimming, kicking, paddling and water running, speed the rehabilitation of injuries, help prevent future injuries, improve general conditioning and help develop specific sport skills. Runners are recognizing that water running, with or without flotation devices, gives a good workout to the muscular and cardiovascular systems while being gentle on the joints.

Resistance work in the water is an excellent way to stay fast, get faster and get strong while reducing the risk of injury. One or two workouts a week, done in the water instead of in your specific sport, may be enough to keep you fresh and injury-free.

MAKE STAYING HEALTHY A HABIT

Eventually, if you stick to a sport long enough, taking care of yourself and staying fit and healthy for competitive events will become almost as important as the training itself. The elements described in this chapter—rest, ice, compression, elevation and hydrotherapy—when approached with an open mind and an ear attentive to the body's needs, are proven methods used by elite and recreational athletes alike to generate personal-best performances. The sooner you come to believe this, the sooner you will be ready to move up another level—no matter who you are.

John Jerome, author of *Staying Supple* and *A Sweet Spot in Time*, defines overuse as "an unfitting level of use," and describes overuse injuries as "our pesky new plague." Jerome says: "To fit the work accurately to the needs of the body may require that we take a little off our level of effort, that we ease up on our determination to always do a bit more." Such backing off may seem heretical to some athletes—the more-is-better crowd—but it represents a logical change in athletic thinking that is bound to produce healthier athletes and better performances at all levels of athletic endeavor. Still, on those inevitable days when limits must be tested and caution thrown to the wind, you can always come home to rest, put out the fire, squeeze the sponge and put up the dogs.

8

STAYING FREE OF INJURY

Such an injury would vex a saint.

WILLIAM SHAKESPEARE, *The Taming of the Shrew*

Staying in shape helps prevent injuries. Yet, anyone who exercises or participates in sports is susceptible to injury. Injuries can occur in any activity, from bullfighting to tiddlywinks. Athletes of all types, from bodybuilders to walkers, limp into doctors' offices with nagging pains, sprains, soreness and inflammation. Many of their problems are avoidable.

With some injuries, the cause is pretty obvious—like when a bike wreck catapults you to the pavement and wrenches your collarbone, or when you land on the side of your ankle after leaping to block a spiked volleyball. But overuse injuries don't announce themselves so dramatically.

An Ounce of Prevention

I remember working on distance runner Craig Virgin at the U.S. Olympic Center in 1989. Craig was having hamstring problems: He had scar tissue built up at the biceps femoris, the main muscle in the hamstring group at the attachment at the buttocks. He was trying to make a comeback into masters' competition to give Bill Rodgers and Frank Shorter a run for their money. But Craig had run for years before massage was prevalent, and he'd done so much damage to his hamstrings over the years that it would have taken years of persistent specialized massage and perhaps medical intervention to clear the problem up. Craig is now a happy recreational runner, but he still has discomfort that I believe could have been prevented had he received massage over the years.

Here are some general rules to help avoid injuries.

Start slowly. The first rule of leading an active life is to get in shape before playing. Experts point out that the highest incidence of injury occurs in the first six to eight weeks of starting an activity or when taking it up again after a period of rest or injury. So begin easily; build up gradually. Increase duration, intensity or resistance by no more than 5 percent per workout. Prevent injuries by careful and faithful preparation through adequate warm-up, warm-down, stretching and massage. Listen to your body and slow down when the sirens begin to whine.

Pay attention to those twinges. Overuse injuries are often sport-specific, resulting from repeated stress to a specific area over a time. We tend to ignore such problems until they become serious. When left unaddressed, healing of overuse injuries can take months or longer. Listening to these signals from your body will enable you to gauge the amount of effort needed in both training and recovery. Learn to speak the body's language, and it will become a partner in the training process. Your body is an intricate feedback mechanism, consciously and unconsciously measuring your level of stress, effort and response.

Know when to back off. In either competition or recovery, the secret in translating the language of the body is knowing when to back off and when to endure. Just as the runner who pushes too hard in the early stages of a race will fade before the finish line, the athlete who trains too hard, too often and without concern for adequate recovery will fade or burn out on a regular basis—usually at the most inconvenient moment. Remember: Your body will warn you before an overuse injury occurs. Listen closely and respond immediately and intelligently.

Give yourself time to recover. When an injury occurs, listen to the body's demands in terms of healing and recovery. When the injury has healed sufficiently, your body will tell you. Be patient. Rush the process, and you may well double your downtime. And take care of all nagging, niggling, annoying physical ailments as soon as you can. True, they may "go away" on their own—at least apparently. But your body never forgets, and you may see those little problems return, maybe bigger and more serious than before, on the most important days in your athletic schedule.

PREVENT INJURY WITH MASSAGE

Injury-free also means "nag-free." As an athlete you should not ignore those little hurts or weaknesses that hinder you just a little bit on a daily basis. If your body is out of tune, it will not perform to its optimum capability—and you'll be asking for more serious injury. Your body doesn't automatically tune itself up, especially if you continue the training that created the problem in the first place.

"If you think of injuries as the result of weaknesses and areas of stress developed over a continuum of time, it is easier to commit to long-term therapy," says Frank Shorter, who won the gold medal in the 1972 Olympic marathon. "I always had the tendency to rehabilitate an injury only to the point where I could resume my pre-injury training intensity. This is what I did from the age of 15 until I turned 35. What I failed to realize was that, by age 35, the accumulated stress of 100 miles per week for decades had resulted in an undetected tightness in my hips and hamstrings." His hips and hamstrings never hurt—just his feet, ankles and back. Today Frank is firmly committed to regular full-body massage. "I deal with this tightness with a regular body massage," he says. "For me the massage is a necessity."

A sensible car owner changes the motor oil before hearing that clattering, screeching sound that says the engine has run dry. That's because the owner keeps track of how many miles the car runs before the oil needs changing. Similarly, a sensible athlete knows how many miles, how many workouts or how many events the body can accommodate before a tune-up becomes necessary. From my work with athletes and my own sports activities, however, I've learned that that level varies greatly from person to person—and that many people ignore the body's demands for "tuning up" even if they do hear them.

Here are a few broad guidelines.

- By the time you feel muscle soreness or strain, you may have already lost precious time that you could have spent in recovery. When you know extra stress has occurred, treat it with massage and rest before it stiffens up.

- In the same way that muscles are more receptive to stretching after training, so, too, are muscles more receptive to stretching following massage. Whenever possible, whether it's training, massage or therapy, stretch afterwards.

- Based on athletes' most commonly reported overuse injuries, the following are areas that all-around athletes should concentrate on during sports massage. (You may want to refer to the illustrations on pages 30 and 31 to check out the muscle groups.)

Feet. In all sports massage, the plantar fascia (connective tissues that create the arch on the bottom of the foot) warrant extra attention. The plantar fascia undergo heavy stresses through repeated pounding from running or constant foot tension created by restrictive footwear worn in sports such as cycling, skating and skiing. Work the length of the tissue, as well as across the grain. Pay close attention to tension or tenderness, working those areas gently until they relax.

Calves and shins. Concentrate on the soleus from the top of the Achilles tendon up to the back of the knee. Do not attempt to massage the Achilles tendon. Visualize the calves in two parts and work upward, dividing the halves with the thumbs. Avoid working the back of the knee. Work up along the shin, as though your fingers could peel the muscle away from the bone. Concentrate on "sticky" or rough spots until they relax.

Quadriceps and iliotibial band. Inflammation of the iliotibial band, known as iliotibial band friction syndrome, can be responsible for knee or hip pain. Tightening of the iliotibial band can also contribute to sideways tracking of the kneecap as the lower leg flexes, causing pain under the kneecap (called patellar compression syndrome). Tight quadriceps can also contribute to both these maladies. Work cross-fiber on the iliotibial band from the knee to the top of the hipbone.

Hamstrings, buttocks and lower back. Hamstrings tend to remain in a semicontracted state, creating an imbalance with the quadriceps. Concentrate on working across the biceps femoris. Work deep through the buttocks to the ball-and-socket joint of the hip, using both the thumb and the elbow techniques.

Upper back, neck and shoulders. The back, neck and shoulders are integral parts of the spinal column and are used in nearly every sport. Relaxing the muscles in this system will benefit the athlete enormously.

Arms and hands. Upper-body athletes such as wrestlers, rock climbers and tennis players will benefit from massage in these areas.

THE MAGIC OF STRETCHING

Stretching can prevent injuries, increase range of motion, restore the length of the muscles to aid in recovery, allow maximal contraction in the next workout and improve biomechanical efficiency. There are several widely accepted and practiced methods of stretching.

Passive stretching. This is done with a partner and involves loosening the tissue surrounding the joint and holding a static or nonmoving stretch for a period of typically 10 to 30 seconds, elongating the muscle by pulling the limb in the opposite direction from which the muscle would move when flexed. The person being stretched can help move the limb, but you gently push to increase the normal range of motion.

Static stretching. Static stretching is the most common method of stretching for athletes. You stretch a muscle slowly to the point of tension, through gravity or manually, and hold it 10 to 30 seconds.

Active stretching. This is a stretch to be done alone, sometimes called dynamic range of motion. It uses antagonistic muscle groups to stretch one another by traversing the natural range of motion in relation to the muscle and the joint. Through this method, you would stretch the hamstring by flexing the quadriceps and hip flexors to extend the hamstring to the limit of its range.

Proprioreceptive neuromuscular facilitation. Also called PNF, this method of stretching is similar to active stretching. It takes advantage of nervous muscle reactions activated by flexion to stretch a particular muscle and needs the cooperation of a partner. Here's an example of how it works.

1. Flex the muscle to be stretched. For example, flex the quadriceps for three to five seconds.

2. Provide a static stretch to the antagonistic muscle group; that is, stretch the hamstring for three to five seconds.

3. Stretch the target area again. (Stretch the quadriceps, for example.)

Ballistic stretching. This is characterized by bouncing or jerking movements and is used by some athletes in the final stages of preparation before competition. This isn't considered a safe form of stretching, however, as you can easily tear or strain muscles by bouncing.

By stretching as a part of warm-up, warm-down and recovery, you may avoid the injuries that plague most athletes. Stretching should be the first response to the minor muscular aches associated with serious exercise. When the body starts talking about the stresses of training, answer first with stretching.

COMBINING STRETCHING AND MASSAGE

To my way of thinking, stretching and massage are closely intertwined; athletes benefit from both. In a logical plan of athletic care and rehabilitation, stretching follows massage and massage follows stretching. One doesn't always have to come first and the other follow, and they don't have to be separate practices. They circle each other, like stars that orbit one another, in an eternally therapeutic ring. To practice only stretching or only massage would leave an athlete incomplete.

LEARN TO TAKE A SNOOZE

This may sound simple, but it's a great injury-prevention tip. Napping is no longer the exclusive domain of kindergartners and those of us trying to avoid Sunday afternoon yard work. Take a nap any time you need it and can fit it in: Science is on your side! According to a Stanford University study, many of us are sleep-deprived. Sleeping for 15 minutes to 2 hours can reduce stress, improve recovery and sharpen mental alertness. We particularly seem to need sleep between midday and early evening.

You may think that napping is wasting time. But the person who is better rested can increase the amount and quality of work accomplished—whether physical effort or mental effort—in less time than the person who is constantly fatigued. Muscle and system recovery are accelerated during sleep, which is why your body needs to sleep in the first place. Remove the distractions associated with consciousness, and the body can get down to the work of serious repair.

History is on the side of the nap indulger: Thomas Edison, Leonardo da Vinci, Amelia Earhart, Thomas Jefferson and Georgia O'Keeffe are among the famous and noteworthy who made napping a part of the day and attribute many of their prodigious talents to this discipline.

As part of athletic recovery, napping is near the top of the list. Because the benefits of napping are in long-term recovery, all short-term treatments should precede the nap. After warm-down, after stretching, after ice and massage and water therapy, then hit the sack. Of course, on the days when you stumble through the door, exhausted and spent, and the only thing your body craves is sleep, waste no time—give the body what it wants!

When you can't keep your thoughts straight or your eyes open, the body is telling you that it has some major repair planned, and it needs the time to do it. Hit the hay. While you snooze, your body will begin the process of transforming you into something new and more powerful.

Stretching a client during a massage is an example of partner-assisted passive stretching, in which an athletic trainer stretches an athlete before the big game. Having completed the soft-tissue massage of an area, it is possible to make use of gentle pulling motions to accentuate the effects of massage by initiating a passive stretch. Experiment with massage and stretching. Try one half of the body, then the other—or finish the entire body's soft-tissue work before beginning the stretching.

Applying mild traction to the neck, fingers, arms and legs is an excellent way to gently stretch during a massage. Pull and shake limbs gently to encourage relaxation of muscles and tissues. Stretch the chest by offering leverage with the arm or perform similar stretches for the hamstrings or quadriceps by using the leg as a lever. By maintaining constant communication with the person you're massaging, you will be able to address the differences and needs of each athlete.

When performing assisted stretches with the person you're massaging, be sure the person is thoroughly warmed up before the stretch. Stretch gently, being constantly aware of the muscle tension, and hold the stretch for 20 to 30 seconds.

Contracted fibers, known as knots, can't be stretched out. Knots will resist stretching through the muscle stretch reflex, holding tighter in response to attempts to stretch the soft tissues. The only reaction to stretching will be further contraction and tighter knots. These fibers are more likely to tear instead of stretch during a sudden stress. These are always the sites of highest likelihood for muscle injury. Massage is probably the best and most accessible means of treating those knots. Stretching following a massage will continue to loosen these knots, and gently massaging the muscle during a stretch will encourage the knot to release.

When massaging yourself, stretch the muscle periodically and concentrate on offering pressure with the hands or an external device such as a massage roller. Incorporating stretching and massage will increase the benefit of both and result in more relaxed, more limber, more quickly recovering athletes capable of performances at higher peaks and increased regularity. Isn't that what every athlete is looking for?

Modern medicine has conditioned us to treat illness rather than wellness. The accepted way has always been to treat ailments after the fact, correcting symptoms but rarely seeking a solution at the source of the trouble. But gradually, athletes have begun to embrace preventive measures such as stretching and massage. By listening to your body and staying one step ahead of its needs, you may lengthen and improve your athletic career.

CHAPTER

9

MASSAGE FOR THE MIND

*Physical exercise is not merely necessary to the health and develop-
ment of the body, but to balance and correct intellectual pursuits as
well. The mere athlete is brutal and Philistine, the mere intellectual
unstable and spiritless. The right education must tune the strings of
the body and mind to perfect spiritual harmony.*

PLATO

To reach the highest levels of performance, the integration of mind and
body is essential. Massage can help balance the body and the mind, but it's only part
of the equation.

Nomadic hunters and gatherers once roamed the land in search of nourish-
ment, often going without food for long periods of time. What kept these nomads
going when they felt fatigued and hopeless?

These days, every year more than 1,500 athletes compete in the Ironman
Triathlon in Hawaii, a modern test of endurance. While training for the Ironman,
triathletes log thousands of miles on a bike, thousands of meters in a pool and thousands of miles on running trails. Then, in one day, finishers endure 8 to 12 hours of

suffering to complete a 2.4-mile swim, a 112-mile bike ride and a 26.2-mile run. Imagine how much intensity it takes to compete in a race like that. What keeps them going?

Well-trained athletes are complete—eating properly, training efficiently, relaxing, getting massages and pursuing other interests besides sport. They are able to balance physical training, mental training, massage, relaxation and rest.

Balance has been determined by many top athletes, including triathlete Mark Allen, as the key to success. Balancing an active lifestyle requires acute awareness of emotional needs, physiological needs and body-awareness needs. To improve athletic performance, the athlete must find a relationship between intensity and relaxation; a perfect union between the body and mind opens the door to peak performances.

The mind needs massage, just like the body.

MENTAL PREPARATION

"Most important, other than training and genetic makeup, is my mental preparation before a major competition," says elite distance runner Arturo Barrios. Two events in particular stand out in his mind as events where his mental preparations were critical: the 10,000 meter race in Berlin and a one-hour run in La Flèche, France—both world record–setting performances.

"Such critical mental preparations can be reached in different ways," he says. "Some people listen to music that will get them motivated for the big race, some people like to read material on various subjects to free their minds from overkill on contemplating the race, and some like to read about performance, competition and the will to win to psych themselves."

The key is to get your mind to work for you, not against you. "The brain can be a tool. It can recall phone numbers, solve math problems or create poetry," writes Dan Mollman in *The Way of the Peaceful Warrior*. "In this way, it works for the rest of the body, like a tractor. But why you can't stop thinking of that math problem or phone number, or when troubling thoughts and memories arise without your intent, it's not your brain working, but your mind wandering. Then the mind controls you; then the tractor has run wild."

The brain is a key function to the pursuit of excellence, in sports and in life. An awareness of how you feel during each stage of competition is crucial. Sports psychologist Kenneth Ravizza of California State University in Fullerton asked several athletes about their experiences with excellence in sport. To no surprise, a wave of common mental factors were retold in interviews. "I was unconscious. Everything was in slow motion. My bike moved around the track effortlessly," said one elite track cyclist.

Pushing the body beyond its limits releases emotion that can affect both audience and performers like a classic Greek drama. When the mind and the body are connected, working together as a unit, a performance can produce a memory that's packed with raw emotion and deep satisfaction. These storage banks of positive emotional states can be used by an athlete to connect the mind with the body.

Drama and competitions have long been linked. Can you have agony without ecstasy? Imagine being at the head of a peloton while bike racing, scaling El Capitan hooked in by carabiners or performing a ballet before hundreds of people. Sports and the intense physical and mental effort they require can influence and motivate an audience. Before he took up triathlons, Mark Allen was watching the Ironman Triathlon on television when he saw competitor Julie Moss stagger and crawl across the finish line. He said to himself, "I have to meet this woman." Mark Allen not only eventually met Julie Moss, but became a top triathlete himself—and the two got married.

HOW TO RELAX YOUR MIND

One of the United States' most successful road cyclists, Davis Phinney, believes that mastering a sport requires total focused concentration, and many athletes would agree. Excellence is a long, grueling process that takes ultimate willpower and devoted commitment—and it takes its toll on both mind and body.

To maintain peak athletic performance, you have to learn to relax. Just as the body needs rest after prolonged intense efforts, the mind experiences similar fatigue after intense levels of concentration and focus.

Skip Hamilton of Aspen, Colorado, is a coach and trainer who works with athletes who compete in cycling, running, cross-country skiing and mountain biking. "We're so steeped in traditional training techniques, we decided to look at mental training and relaxation techniques," he says. "We've overlooked balancing intensity with relaxation techniques like yoga, stretching and sports massage. Calming the mind with relaxation responses allows us to go harder. . . . Peak performance, those unleashed events we dream about, can be achieved! These same processes happen every day to the non-elite athlete who is in pursuit of excellence."

Meditation, breathing and visualization are techniques that allow the mind to focus when it needs to and let go when it doesn't. Other methods of relaxation include acupuncture, yoga, reiki, Zen and Rolfing. These methods can enhance the quality of physical training by placing the mind and body in a state of readiness to compete.

Here are some tips to help you relax and take a step toward achieving the balance of body, mind and spirit that an athlete needs to succeed.

Analyze your life and your training tactics. Ask yourself: What five things are stopping me from feeling good about my lifestyle and my training? What can I change? What things are blocking a positive attitude? Am I overtraining? Am I taking enough time to balance an active lifestyle?

Visit people who speak your language. You can draw inspiration and motivation from people with similar pursuits and dreams. In Boulder, where I live and work, you can always find athletes hanging around local coffee shops discussing related ideas about their sports, which often leads to a positive, motivated sense of self. Such environments—shops that sell cycling, skiing, climbing or other kinds of equipment, even monthly club meetings or magazines—can be exciting and stimulating.

Practice relaxation. You may think that lying around or talking with friends is relaxing, but chances are your mind is still cluttered and parts of your body are tense. Set aside 15 to 30 minutes for deliberate relaxation. Choose a darkened, quiet room, then make yourself comfortable and clear your mind by thinking of a relaxing scene, such as waves rolling onto the beach or a lone hawk circling in the sky. Breathe slowly and deeply, and then deliberately tense and then relax each set of muscles in turn. You may want to pick serene music to help, or try a relaxation tape.

Stick to calming rituals. For many people, a specific routine is calming, particularly prior to competition. You may want to listen to certain music, read a book, do a set of stretches or put on your "lucky" pair of socks. Do whatever works for you.

Sample this menu of tips. Try some of these ideas to help yourself relax.

- Take time out just for yourself.

- Visit a place that mentally stimulates you, such as a bookstore or a museum.

- Practice yoga or tai chi.

- Spend time with family and friends.

- Leave some unscheduled time during your day.

- Go to bed early enough to get the amount of sleep that you need.

THE VALUE OF VISUALIZATION AND MENTAL IMAGERY

"Doing visualization should be a daily routine," says Skip Hamilton. When athletes engage in visualization, they temporarily change their environments. This can be used to relax the mind and body or to practice skills. Visualization activates the neural pathways as if they were processing the information of actual experiences. This literally permits the creation of alternative events and the learning of new skills. The nervous system cannot distinguish an imagined from a real experience.

Gymnasts will review their routines hundreds of times before they perform.

Baseball players visualize hitting a ball before it is hit. Cyclists review a race by seeing the road surface and knowing what gears they will be using. To be in a zone of focused concentration, an athlete must be properly prepared.

It's best to use this method before a competition. However, it is also helpful after competition to work out weaknesses and improve technique. These methods can be incorporated into giving and receiving massage, enhancing performance and improving concentration. Visualize the entire race from start to finish. Take your time in seeing the picture unfold.

Here are four steps to effective visualization.

- Relax with a massage. Lie down and become aware of physical tension. Let go of tensions by concentrating on specific body parts that are tight. Gently flex the muscle group that is holding tension, then slowly relax it. Do this with every body part. Imagine a peaceful scene—the quiet warmth and solitude of a sunny secluded beach, for example.

- Remember a successful scene from the past. Recall every detail of the most positive, invigorating experience that you have ever had. Hear the screaming fans. Enjoy the looks of admiration from spectators and friends as they congratulate you. Revel in the praise from coaches and fellow competitors. Concentrate on the feeling of pride as you receive your award and relate the event to reporters.

- Substitute an imagined situation of the future for the recollection of a past experience. Replace the past exciting experience with the accomplishment of goals. Do not fear the goals that enter your imagination that may not seem realistic. Let your imagination run wild. Albert Einstein said that his most important insights were achieved through images. He first realized the distortion of time and space by imagining riding on a beam of the sun traveling at the speed of light.

- Use every sense to visualize. For example, a diver must recall not only the smell of chlorine but also the feel of the diving board, the taste of water and the sounds around the pool. You must use as many senses as possible. The more detail you can recall, the more effective the visual-ization. The emotions of various sport experiences are also very important for effective visualization.

Kim Isherwood, a professional triathlete who lives in Hong Kong, said, two days before the New Zealand Ironman, "I really get relaxed. I see it; feel it; and I rewind the tape one or two times. In training, I get feedback. I visualize: This is how it will feel out there."

. . . .

WHERE TO LEARN MORE

There are many other types of bodywork, many of which involve the mind as well as the body. Here's some background information on a variety of techniques.

Rolfing. Rolfing, based on the concept that you function better both mentally and physically when your body is properly aligned, was developed by biochemist Ida Rolf, Ph.D. Over ten sessions, Rolfing works on a deep level to free fascia on all parts of the body to improve structural alignment. Muscles that have become chronically tight from training, injury, emotional blocks or physical tension can be released through this technique to increase freedom of movement and range of motion. From my own experience as an athlete and professional bodyworker, I find this most effective during the off-season, when the body has more time to recover from the deep-tissue work. Contact the Rolf Institute, 302 Pearl Street, Boulder, CO 80302; (303) 449-5903.

Aston-Patterning. Judith Aston, a student of Ida Rolf, believed that some asymmetry in the body is normal. Aston-Patterning, a variation of Rolfing, takes into account individual differences among people and focuses on changing only unnatural asymmetry. This type of bodywork can help you develop three-dimensional movement awareness through deep massage. Contact the Aston Training Center, Box 3568, Incline Village, NV 89450; (702) 831-8228.

Hellerwork. Joseph Heller, also a student of Ida Rolf, came up with an offshoot of Rolfing using deep-tissue bodywork to improve structural integration through verbal and video feedback. Contact Hellerwork, Inc., 406 Berry Street, Mount Shasta, CA 96067; 1-800-392-3900.

Alexander Technique. F. M. Alexander was a late twentieth–century actor

. . . .

PUTTING IT ALL TOGETHER

So now it's race day, and you want to do your best. See your sport environment from the minute you wake. Close your eyes and begin by focusing on your breathing. Let the tensions of daily activities go with each breath.

Go to a special place in your mind: Imagine a room where you can be at peace and comfortable in your mind and surrounded by things that please you.

who developed a technique to overcome poor posture habits that interfere with coordination and performance. The Alexander Technique for athletes is designed to reduce incorrect repetitive motion that leads to injury and can teach you how to move in better harmony with your body, increasing your sense of ease and performance. Contact the North American Society of Teachers of the Alexander Technique, Box 517, Urbana, IL 61801; 1-800-473-0629.

Feldenkrais Method. Moshe Feldenkrais was an Israeli physicist and athlete who discovered that the brain sends messages to the body about how we move. If a particular movement causes recurring injuries, the body can help the brain repattern itself and eliminate deeply embedded patterns of tension and, therefore, the outward signs of injury. Contact the Feldenkrais Guild, Box 489, Albany, OR 97321; 1-800-775-2118.

Pilates Method. Joseph Pilates was a German dancer who developed a system to condition an athlete for muscle strength and flexibility. The Pilates Method incorporates dance training principles and is intended to increase body awareness and enhance coordination. Contact the Institute for Pilates, 1807 Second Street, Unit 28, Santa Fe, NM 87501; (505) 988-1990

Trager Work. Developed by Milton Trager, M.D., in the 1920s, this is a gentle, rhythmic rocking and stretching designed to subconsciously break up old tension patterns. Trager Work encourages deep relaxation and improves mental clarity. I like to use this technique a day or two before a major race or as a change of pace from regular massage. Contact the Trager Institute, 33 Millwood, Mill Valley, CA 94941; (415) 388-2688.

Review the equipment you will be using and your clothing. See yourself warming up and allow your body to get ready to perform.

See and feel your competitors. Realize that you have had proper training. Focus the mind on what your body needs to do. Be your own guide. Review your plan and look for mistakes or anything you have forgotten.

Review the conditions: See the road surface, feel the snow or the glare of the sun. Notice the new sights, listen to the sounds, smell the air. Sense the emotion associated with finishing well. See and feel yourself performing a skill in slow motion. Allow the mind to let go of negative images. Focus on positive images and draw from past mental images.

You want to arrive at the start at a calm level of intensity. You need to experiment to find out what works for you. It may be listening to tapes of Jimi Hendrix or Enya or reading poetry.

Ask yourself these questions.

- Have I prepared physically and mentally for this event?

- Do I control my actions?

- Can I feel my muscles relax?

- Can I feel my blood flow?

- Can I see and feel myself doing a skill without a mistake?

Whether it's competing in the giant slalom or making a key presentation to a major corporation, the first step is preparing the mind and the body to act together. Plan ahead of time: Schedule your massage 36 hours before an important event to allow the blood time to circulate properly. Practice your visualization techniques well before the competition. Leave early for your event and (naturally) take the weather into consideration. Now, rest assured that you are ready to compete and put your abilities on the line. You've taken a huge step toward preparing body and mind to work together to produce an optimum performance.

10

WHAT THE ATHLETES SAY

Success rests in having the courage and endurance and, above all, the will to become the person you are. However peculiar that may be, then you will be able to say 'I have found my hero, and he is me.'

GEORGE SHEEHAN, M.D., RUNNER'S WORLD

Have any lingering doubts about the value of massage? The best people to explain the value of sports massage are athletes—the people who spend huge chunks of their lives participating in sports to the utmost of their abilities.

In the course of writing this book, I sent questionnaires to athletes and clients asking them to outline their impressions of massage. Among the questions I asked were "How have massage and self-massage contributed to your training and competition?" and "What do you do to enhance recovery and rest periods?"

Here's what they had to say.

MARK ALLEN: A CONVERT TO MASSAGE

Mark Allen is a four-time winner of the Hawaii Ironman Triathlon.

People often overlook one of the most important elements of any training program: recovery. Aspects of this unsung hero range from a good diet to high-tech gadgetry designed to realign your body's energy fields. I've tried almost everything out there, and I always come back to one of the oldest and simplest modalities to keep my weary bones running fast and my tired muscles supple and injury-free: good old hands-on massage.

When I started triathlons in 1982, I'd never received a massage. After a buddy suggested that it would help my recovery and performance, I went—with skepticism in hand. After five massages five weeks in a row, I said 'enough'—and began to realize how truly important massage is.

My training had been coming along really well those five weeks. I thought my quicker recovery rate and reduced aches and pains were because I was getting in shape. But after missing several massages, my recovery rate was sluggish and those nagging aches were back. I realized that greater sense of well-being had come from massage.

In the more than a dozen years since, massage has become an indispensable part of my training and recovery program. I've traveled the world as a triathlete and at every important race, the gentleman who gave me that first massage has been there to make sure that my body is ready to perform at its best.

Not that massage is a cure-all. You need to be sensible in your training and about who you choose to work on your body. All massage therapists bring their own interpretations of standard techniques to the work. They all have a different "feel." Your choice of a therapist is as important as your choice of friends. Be willing to experiment with more than one person and to ask for different types of work from the same person. The exact same massage each time is like eating the exact same dish for dinner each night. Your body's needs and appetites change, and it's up to you to have a good enough relationship with your therapist to figure out what it is that you need.

Just as nothing replaces the hard work that an athlete must do to perform, nothing replaces massage as a tool for enhancing recovery rate, preventing injuries and reducing stress.

ARTURO BARRIOS: LISTEN TO YOUR BODY

Arturo Barrios held the world record in the 10,000 meters (27:08:23) from August 1989 until July 1993. Shortly after taking up the marathon, he ran a 2:08:28 at Boston in 1994 and finished third in the 1994 New York City Marathon.

Staying healthy and uninjured isn't easy when you're asking your body to perform at peak levels throughout most of each year. You need to have everything in your favor, and that means enhancing recovery by any means possible. Massage is one of the ways that helps me avoid injury. Getting massaged at least once a week will help prevent all types of injuries, including injuries to the knee, Achilles tendon, hamstring, calf, back and even neck. I try to get massaged twice a week because it helps me recover quickly from track workouts. I find that this regular bodywork loosens up my muscles, reduces stress and permits me to keep motivated for the next day's workout.

Remember: In order to remain consistent in your training and constant in your progress toward long-term goals, you must stay healthy and uninjured. It is vital to maintain good habits. You must also listen to your body, which is your best doctor. When you experience pain, your body is trying to tell you something. Usually it's overuse, but it might also be a biomechanical problem developing. You may find it necessary to consult a massage therapist who specializes in neuromuscular therapy. Quick recovery from any problem is vital in maintaining the consistency and progress necessary for success.

SALLY EDWARDS: "JUST FEEL IT"

Endurance athlete Sally Edwards of Sacramento holds the Ironman Masters' World Record, won the 1980 Western States 100-Mile Endurance Run and participated in the 1984 Olympic Marathon Trials. Sally is also the founder of Fleet Feet stores and the author of eight books on triathlons and fitness.

When I first met Joan Johnson, I was not a big advocate of massage; I felt it was but a minor player in the complicated equation of successful athletic training and competition. And I didn't want to deal with the time and cost of regular visits to a massage therapist.

Now I know I was wrong. Joan has shown me that even for someone with a busy travel schedule and a diverse professional life, massage should be a high priority. When I'm in the office for hours, I practice self-massage and use massage devices. That empowers me: I'm literally able to take into my own hands the relief and therapy my working muscles sorely need.

When I'm preparing for a race, I use techniques that link mind and body. People tend to embrace the Nike slogan of "Just Do It," but I encourage a more personal philosophy of "Just Feel It." I listen closely to my body to hear those areas that need attention, then I respond quickly with sports massage.

Massage is especially important when you're asking your body to perform again and again at peak levels. During one three-month period, I competed in four Ironman-length triathlons and attempted to set the masters' world record in each. I had to keep extending my conditioning while staying injury-free. Sports massage helped me find my weak areas and rehabilitate them, find areas of imbalance and recondition them and find areas of power and support them.

Your ability to know yourself and then use that knowledge to coach yourself can help you achieve a lifetime of training and racing. Fitness is a higher form of health. Massage helps me achieve that higher form by promoting balance and self-esteem in body and mind.

ROBYN ERBESFIELD: CUTS DOWN RECOVERY TIME

Robyn Erbesfield is a world-champion rock climber who lives part of the year in France and part in Boulder. She placed first in the 1992 World Cup series.

I'm a firm believer in massage therapy, not only for athletes but for anyone suffering from stress, strain or fatigue. While it's important to massage specific areas that are stressed, it's perhaps more important to have a massage regularly to avoid the stress and strain of everyday activities, especially sports.

I get a massage once or twice a week. Massage is for me a method of recuperating and rejuvenating that can replace a rest day or two, which would inhibit my long-term training results. In essence, massage allows me to recover more rapidly than a full rest day. When I do take a rest day, I like to stretch, go for a light run and relax during a full body massage.

My schedule leading up to an event is often stress-filled, not only because of the intense training but also because of anxiety about a certain competition. I've found that massage therapy allows me to relax all my muscles and visualize myself being fit and ready—either for the competition or another training day.

WES HOBSON: MASSAGE IS A "FOURTH SPORT"

Wes Hobson of Boulder, Colorado, was named 1992 Male Triathlete of the Year by the United States Olympic Committee. In 1993 he was fourth overall in the International Triathlon Union World Cup series, and he led off the 1994 season with a victory at a World Cup race in Amakusa, Japan.

Massage helps me maintain muscle coordination, improve flexibility and prevent injuries. My favorite time for a massage is late afternoon, after training, especially after a swim workout. Then my body is tired, yet relaxed, and it's more willing to let the massage therapist into deeper sections of muscle without tensing up. I like to visualize the therapist taking the muscle from the body and "tenderizing" it like meat. I visualize how the therapist is breaking up tightly bound muscle, ridding it of lactic acid and stretching and lengthening it to improve flexibility.

Find a competent massage therapist who works on you regularly. This way the therapist knows your body and your problem spots. Even so, it is important to communicate with your therapist and tell them what areas need most work. They can't always feel the stressed areas. That's one reason self-massage is particularly valuable: No one knows your body like you do. My best times to self-massage are while watching TV or in the sauna or hot tub after workouts. Plane trips are also good; you're confined to one area and there are no urges to do errands or household chores.

If I were to have three wishes in life, one would be to have a two-hour massage every day. Maybe in heaven.

KIM JONES: PART OF A FITNESS REGIMEN

Kim Jones of Spokane was the number-one ranked American marathoner in 1986, 1989 and 1991. Her personal best of 2:26:40, set in the 1991 Boston Marathon, is the fourth fastest U.S. performance of all time.

For maybe the first five years that I was running, I didn't use massage. I was mostly injury-free, and I just didn't think I needed to do anything other than train and rest.

I started having problems, though, after I blistered badly running the 1990 Boston Marathon. The blisters caused me to alter my form. That's when I decided to try massage. It helped, and I became a believer.

After I began having regular massages, I became aware of how much they benefited my running overall. Massage helped me recover more quickly from hard workouts. And I've found it helps prevent injury. My massage therapist knows when any of my muscles are tight or just "off" a little. She works on it right away; that prevents it from becoming a problem.

I also have my therapist do what's called fascia release about once every two weeks. She may begin working on my quads, then another part of my body will begin to burn or feel tight or ache, so she moves on to that. Basically, my body directs her where to work next. It's a relaxing type of massage, and I have a great workout the next day.

I've begun using self-massage as well. I was hit by a bicycle while running, and I pulled my right calf. I began to use self-massage—along with ice and my standard massage—and the injury has been getting better.

I've told people, mostly jokingly, that a pot of coffee is my most important pre-race strategy. But I also switch to a slightly different type of massage, called soma or somassage, which is a combination of sports massage and fascia release. Three firm strokes are applied to each muscle group, not so much digging into the muscle as going over it.

So for me, massage is an important part of an overall training program that includes, among other things, stretching, ice, naturopathic gels and creams and attention to diet. Using these techniques keeps me healthy. Of course, I also have to avoid stepping on large objects in the middle of the road.

JANE McCONNELL: TRAINING FOR MOTHERHOOD

Jane McConnell is publisher and editor-in-chief of Women's Sports and Fitness *magazine. She's also a marathoner, cyclist, skier, kayaker and mother.*

As my massage therapist, Joan was one of the first people outside my family to learn that I was pregnant. Massage has always been an emotional as well as a physical therapy for me. Lying on the massage table the day I told her, I was able to let go of both muscle tension and my anxiety surrounding this new development.

Massage soothed me through each stage of my first pregnancy. In the beginning, it relieved the unfamiliar emotional and physical sensations I was experiencing. As an athlete, it was hard for me not to think of my pregnancy as an injury that slowed me down and limited my activity. I felt sick to my stomach, couldn't sleep well and experienced wild mood swings. Throughout it all, massage was an oasis of calm.

As my baby grew, so did my excitement. I wanted to do everything I could to take care of the two of us. Massage got my blood circulating to nourish the baby and worked from my back and legs the soreness caused by carrying extra weight.

Once I felt better, I was able to keep up regular exercise and began exploring sports new to me, like swimming and yoga. I continued to cycle ten miles to and from work each day and to take long hikes with my dogs. Massage kept me injury-free, and that's especially important for pregnant women.

With the birth imminent, I continued regular massage. Joan devised an egg carton–style foam pad with a hole cut in it so I could lie comfortably on my stomach. While I felt heavy and ungainly on my feet, the massage table allowed me to let go. The baby seemed to enjoy it too, responding with happy little movements.

As I prepared for the most important athletic event of my life, massage was a crucial part of my training.

JOHN TEAFORD: HOW TO FIGHT OFF INJURIES

John Teaford is an international speed skating competitor and former coach of the United States Speed Skating Team.

Over the years, the one constant I've come to recognize in athletics is that you don't have to feel good to "go" good. Depending on how good I feel as a prerequisite for good performance would amount to limiting myself mentally every time I stepped up to the starting line. So I judge sport, body and fitness exclusively by finishing time and try to ignore the "feel." I rely on history for my proof—and on massage for my therapy.

Although I trust in the healing that massage offers me, I don't approach the table with ease. The first minutes are always a struggle as my squirming, resisting muscles awake in tiny spasms and ticklish fear. Other people I know come home from massage raving about how much better they feel. Either I'm totally out of touch with my body, or I never feel that bad to begin with. I come home knowing only that massage has helped me prepare for a performance superior to what I would have had without it.

My 33-year-old body twists through workouts designed for younger hips, straighter backs and smoothly functioning knees. Little injuries, sore spots and weak links threaten daily to drag me further down the path of diminishing performance. But as yet, no ailment has been smarter than me—or beyond the reach of my massage therapist's fingers. I cannot imagine an injury that would not get better if treated with massage.

INDEX

Note: Underscored page references indicate boxed text.
Boldface references indicate illustrations.

A

Abdomen massage, 62, **62–64**
Achilles tendon, **48**
Active stretching, 139
Acupressure, 4, 28
Acupuncture, 4
Acu-Reflex Massager, 22
Adductor muscles, **78**
Adhesions, 25
Aerobic exercise, glycogen depletion from, 132
Alexander, F. M., 148–49
Alexander technique, 148–49
Allen, Mark, 144, 145, 152
Allergies, to lubricants, 19
Almond oil, for massage, 18
American Massage Therapy Association
    (AMTA), 4, 5, 73
Ankle massage, 49, **49–50**
Anterior deltoid muscle, **81**
Arches of feet, massaging, **61**, **76**
Arm massage
    concentration areas in, 138
    self-massage, **81**
    techniques, 64, **65–66**
Aromatherapy, 19
Arthritis, therapists' development of, 10
Aston, Judith, 148
Aston-Patterning, 148
Aston Training Center, 148

Athletes. *See also specific names*
    self-massage and, views of, 151–57
    sports massage and
        use of, 1–2, 5
        views of, 151–57
    tenderness near knee and, **53**
Avocado oil, for massage, 18

B

Baby oil, for massage, 18
Back massage
    concentration areas in, 138
    lubricants for, 34
    self-massage, 80, **84–85**
    techniques, 34, **34–41**
Backpacking sports massage techniques, 101,
    102–3, 103
Ballistic stretching, 139
Barrios, Arturo, 1, 128, 144, 152–53
Better Back Store, The, 22
Biathletes, 115–16
Biceps, **81**, 123
Bicycling sports massage techniques
    mountain biking, 105, **105–7**
    road biking, 92, **93–94**, 95
Biofeedback, from self-massage, 76
Bioscape Mattress Pads, 22
Biotone, 18, 20

Body
    asymmetry in, 148
    awareness of, massage and, 3
    as guide for massaging techniques, 29–31
    listening to, 132, 136, 152–53
    meridians, 28
    position, for massaging clients, 17
    temperature, during massage, 14
    weight, in supplementing hand pressure, 10
Bodybuilding sports massage techniques, 95
Breathing
    of receivers of massage, 31
    of therapists, during massage, 17, 29, 31, **61**
Buttocks massage
    concentration areas in, 138
    self-massage, **80**, **86**
    techniques, 42, **42–43**

C

Calf massage
    concentration areas in, 138
    self-massage, **77**
    techniques, **44**, **47–48**
Carbohydrates, diet high in, 132
Carpal tunnel syndrome, of therapists, 10
Chest massage
    self-massage, **82**, **85**
    techniques, 62, **62–64**
Chondromalacia patellae, 101
Circulation problems, massage for, 49
"Climber's wrist," 107
Climbing sports massage techniques, 107,
    108–9, 109
Coconut oil, for massage, 18
Colorado Healing Arts Products, 17
Communication in massage, 10
Competition
    listening to body during, 136
    mind massage and, 148–50
Compression methods, 23, 130
Coogan, Gwyn, 29–30, 32
Cooldowns, massage during, 95
Court sports, 95
    sports massage techniques, 95, **96–98**, 98
Creams, hand, 9–10. *See also* Lubricants
Cross-country skiing sports massage techniques,
    115–16
Cross-fiber stroking, 26, **46**, **48**, **57**, **77**, **78**, **80**
Cross-training techniques, 3, 32, 91
Cupping in tapotement massage technique, 27, **27**
Curative/restorative massage, 32
Cycling. *See* Bicycling sports massage techniques

D

Deep-tissue massage, 28, 29, **36**, **45**
Deep transverse friction. *See* Cross-fiber
    stroking
Deltoid muscles, **81**, 123
Diet, recovery from hard effort and, 132
Dietary fat, diet low in, 132
Downhill skiing sports massage techniques, 116,
    117–19
Draining-the-arm technique, **66**, **67**
Dual-Purpose Massage Creme, 18

E

Ears, tugging on during facial massage, **71**
Edwards, Sally, 153–54
Effleurage massage technique, 25, **26**, **34**, **44**,
    47, **57**
Elevation methods, 131
Erbesfield, Robyn, 107, 109, 154
Essences, for sports massage, 19
Essential oils, for sports massage, 19
Ethafoam cylinder, 84. *See also* Massage Roller
Everybody, Ltd., 20
Eyes
    massaging around, **71**
    placing hands over, at end of massage, **72**

F

Face cradle, on massage table, 15
Facial massage, **71–72**
Fat, diet low in, 132
Feet. *See* Foot massage
Feldenkrais, Moshe, 149
Feldenkrais Guild, 149
Feldenkrais method, 149
Field sports, 95
    sports massage techniques, 95, **96–98**, 98
Finger board, 8–9, **9**
Fingers
    feel for massage in, developing, 12
    pulling on, in hand massage, **68**
    strengthening exercises for, 7–9, **8**, **9**
    stretching, **8**
Fitness, physical, 135, 136, 155
Floor, as work surface for massage, 14
Flu, avoiding massage after, 33
Fluids, replenishing after exercise, 132
Foam Roller Therapy, 84
Foot Massage (product), 22

Foot massage
    ankles, 49, **49–50**
    arches, **61**, **76**
    back of, 41, **51–52**
    concentration areas in, 137–38
    flexing foot and, **50**
    front of, 59, **59–61**
    plantar fascia, 138
    pressure of massage in, **60**
    sand as therapeutic medium for, 122
    self-massage, **76**
    soles, **51**
    stretching foot and, 59
Forearm self-massage techniques, **81**
Friction massage technique, 26, **26**, 29, **36**
Frostbite, avoiding during ice massage, 130

G

Glycogen, depletion of, 132
Golden Ratio Woodworks, 17
Golf sports massage techniques, 99–100, **99–100**
Gymnastics sports massage techniques, 100–101

H

Hacking in tapotement massage technique, 27, **28**
Hamilton, Skip, 145
Hamstring massage
    concentration areas in, 138
    self-massage, **79**, **86–87**
    techniques, 44, **44–48**
Hands
    body weight to supplement pressure of, 10
    caring for, 9–10
    client's response with, gauging, 10
    concentration areas in massage of, 138
    creams for, 9–10
    endurance of, in massaging, 7
    finger-strengthening exercises and, 7–9, **8**, **9**
    hydrotherapy for, 10
    lotions for, 9–10
    massage techniques for, 64, **65–69**
    relaxation of, 11
    self-massage, **76**
Hansen, Eric, 119
Hard effort, signs of, 128. *See also* Recovery
        from hard effort
Head massage, 70, **70–72**
Heart, stroking toward, 29
Heller, Joseph, 148
Hellerwork, 148
Hellerwork, Inc., 148

Herbal lubricants, 19
Hiking sports massage techniques, 101, **102–3**, 103
Hobson, Wes, 154–55
Hydration, for recovery from hard effort, 132
Hydrotherapy, 10, 131–33, 140

I

Ice massage, 101, 129–30, 140
Ice therapy, traditional, 10, 128, 129
Iliotibial band
    inflammation of, 105, 138
    self-massage, **88**
    soreness, 101, 105
Iliotibial band friction syndrome, 138
Inflammation, 129
    of iliotibial band, 105, 138
    of patellar tendons, 101
Injuries. *See also specific types*
    cautions for massage use with, 33
    from overuse, 2, 122, 133, 136
    prevention of, 136–37
        cross-training techniques and, 91
        fitness and, physical, 135, 136
        ice massage in, 130
        massage and, 42, **54**, **56**, 64, 91
        massage-stretching combination and, 139, 141
        napping and, 140
        sports massage and, 1–2, 5, 137–38, 139,
            141, 156–57
        strengthening exercises and, 92
        stretching and, 92, 138–39, 141
    running, 101, 109–10
    swimming, 119
    treatment of, with massage, 2–3
Institute for Pilates, 149
Isherwood, Kim, 147–48

J

Joints, surgery on, **58**
Jones, Kim, 131, 155
Joyner-Kersee, Jackie, 5

K

Kayaking sports massage techniques, 103, **104**, 105
Kellogg, John H., 4
Kneecap
    massage techniques, 56, **56**
    pain under, 138
    softening of, 101

Knee massage, 56, **56**
Knobble, 22
Knots, in muscles, **40**, 141

L

Lactic acid, cleansing from body, 129
Latissimus dorsi muscle, 27, **82**
Leg massage
    back of, 42, **43**
    calves, **44**, **47–48**
    front of, 52, **52–55**
    hamstrings, 44, **44–48**
    knees, 56, **56**
    quadriceps, **53**, 57, **57–58**
    shins, **53–55**
LeMond, Greg, 5, 92
Lifestyle, healthy, 133, 144
Ligaments, 42
Lighting during massage, 14
Ling, Per Henrick, 4
Living Earth Crafts, 17
Lockyer, Roch, 92
Lotions, hand, 9–10. *See also* Lubricants
Lubricants
    allergies to, 19
    for back massage, 34
    cautions in using, 19, 20
    in curative/restorative massage, 32
    in foot massage, 51
    herbal, 19
    in post-event massage, 32
    during pregnancy, use of, 19
    scented, 19
    skin's cooling and, 14, 32
    sources for buying, 20
    as tool for massage, 17–18, 19, 20

M

McConnell, Jane, 156
McKenzie, Tait, 4
Massage. *See also* Sports massage; Techniques,
        massage
    balance of body and mind and, 143
    body awareness and, 3
    cautions in giving or receiving, 33
    for circulation problems, 49
    communication in, 10
    during cooldowns, 95
    discomfort after, 10
    ending, **72**
    history of, 3–5
    injuries and
        prevention of, 42, **54**, **56**, 64, 91
        treatment of, 2–3
    lighting during, 14
    mental imaging during, 11
    mood during, 20–21
    muscles and, 12
    music during, 20–21
    non-sports, 2, 3–5
    outdoor, 14
    pain after, 10
    during pregnancy, 33
    recovery from hard effort and, 128–29
    regular, 2, 3–5
    relaxation and, 2
    rest and, 128
    room used for, 14
    schools, 73
    setting of, 14
    spontaneity in, 11–12
    stretching in combination with, 139, 141
    table, self-made, 16
    visualization during, 11
    work surfaces for, 14–15
Massage parlors, 4
Massage Roller
    hiking/backpacking sports massage techniques
        with, 101, **102–3**
    self-massage with, 84, **84–89**
    sources for buying, 84
Massage Store, Ltd., The, 20, 22, 84
Massage tools, 21–23, 83–84. *See also specific
        types*
Mental alertness, napping in sharpening, 140
Mental imagery
    during massage, 11
    in mind massage, 146–48
Meridians, body, 28
Milking-the-arm technique, **66**, **67**
Mind-body improvement techniques,
        148–49
Mind massage
    Alexander technique and, 148–49
    Aston-Patterning and, 148
    competition and, 148–50
    Feldenkrais method and, 149
    Hellerwork and, 148
    importance of, 143–44
    mental imagery in, 146–48
    mental preparation for, 144–47
    Pilates method and, 149

relaxation and, 145–46
Rolfing and, <u>148</u>
Trager work and, <u>149</u>
visualization in, 146–48
Mineral oil, for massage, 18
Mood during massage, 20–21
Moss, Julie, 145
Mountain biking sports massage techniques,
     105, **105–7**
Mountain climbing sports massage techniques,
     107, **108–9**, 109
Muscles. *See also* Hamstring massage; Quadricep
     massage
  adductor, **78**
  anterior deltoid, **81**
  biceps, **81**, 123
  chest, 62
  contracted fibers in, 141
  deltoid, **81**, 123
  groups of, **30**, **31**
  after hard effort, 128
  knots in, **40**, 141
  latissimus dorsi, 27, **82**
  ligaments, 43
  massage and, 12
  microtears in, 2, 129
  overuse of, 2, 133, 136
  pectoralis major and minor, **82**
  recovery from hard effort and, 128, <u>132</u>
  during rest, 128
  Rolfing and, 29
  soleus, 138
  sore, 31, 116
  sports massage and, 2–3, <u>2</u>, 29
  under stress, 130
  tendons, 43
  trapezius, 27, **82**
  triceps, 27, **81**, 123
Music during massage, 20–21

N

Nails (of therapist), caring for, 10
Napping, for injury prevention, <u>140</u>
Neck massage
  concentration areas in, 138
  self-massage, **82**
  techniques, 70, **70–72**
Nelson, Lyle, 115–16
Non-sports massage, <u>2</u>, 3–5. *See also* Massage
North American Society of Teachers of the
     Alexander Technique, <u>149</u>

O

Oakworks, Inc., 17
Oils. *See* Lubricants
Outdoor massage, 14
Overtraining, recognizing signs of, 32
Overuse injuries, 2, 122, 133, 136

P

Passive stretching, 138–39
Patella
  massage and, 56, **56**
  pain under, 138
  softening of, 101
Patellar compression syndrome, 138
Patellar tendinitis, 101
Peach oil, for massage, 18
Pectoralis major and minor muscles, **82**
Petrissage massage technique, 27, **27**, 29, **41**
Pilates, Joseph, <u>149</u>
Pilates method, <u>149</u>
Plaatjes, Mark, 29
Plantar fascia, massage of, 138
PNF stretching, 139
Position of therapist in massage, 11, 14–16, 17
Post-event massage, 32
Pre-event massage, 32
Pregnancy
  lubricant use during, <u>19</u>
  massage during, <u>33</u>
  sports massage during, 156
Pressure of massage
  on back of knee, avoiding, **46**, **48**
  body weight to supplement hand, 10
  comfortable, 11
  experimenting with, 11
  in foot massage, **60**
  increasing, 31
  in trigger-point therapy, 28
Pro Massage Company, 83
Proprioreceptive neuromuscular facilitation
     (PNF) stretching, 139
Protein, diet high in, <u>132</u>

Q

Quadricep massage
  concentration areas in, 138
  self-massage, **78**, **88**
  techniques, **53**, 57, **57–58**

R

Ravizza, Kenneth, 144
Recovery from hard effort
  compression methods and, 130
  diet and, 132
  elevation methods and, 131
  hydration and, 132
  hydrotherapy and, 131–33
  ice massage and, 129–30
  lifestyle and, healthy, 133
  massage and, 128–29
  muscles and, 128, 132
  quick, 127–28
  rest and, 128–29, 140
  sleeping and, 128–29, 140
  sports massage and, 154
  stretching and, 139
  time allotted for, 136–37
  water massage and, 131–33
Reflexology, 29, 51
Regular massage, 2, 3–5. *See also* Massage
Relaxation, 145–46
  baths for, after massaging clients, 10
  breathing for, before massaging clients, 17
  of hands, 11
  massage and, 2
  mind massage and, 145–46
  music and, 20–21
  practicing, 146
  rituals and, calming, 146
  sports massage and, 113
  of therapists, during massage, 11, 31
Resistance work in water, 133
Rest, recovery from hard effort and, 128–29, 140
RICE (rest, ice, compression and elevation), 128
Rituals, calming, 146
Rock climbing sports massage techniques, 107, **108–9**, 109
"Rocking Horse" stroke, **38**
Rolf, Ida, 29, 148
Rolfing, 29, 148
Rolf Institute, 148
Room used for massage, 14
Rotation of ankle, **49**
Rowing sports massage techniques, 103, **104**, 105
Runner's knee, 101
Running
  injuries, 101, 109–10
  sports massage techniques, 109–10, **110–12**
  trail, 101

S

Salves. *See* Lubricants
Schools, massage, 73
SelfCare Catalog, 23
Self-massage techniques
  arms, **81**
  athletes' views of, 151–57
  back, **80**, **84–85**
  benefits of, 75–76
  biofeedback from, 76
  buttocks, **80**, **86**
  calves, **77**
  chest, **82**, **85**
  feet, **76**
  forearms, **81**
  hamstrings, **79**, **86–87**
  hands, **76**
  iliotibial band, **88**
  with Massage Roller, 84, **84–89**
  neck, **82**
  quadriceps, **78**, **88**
  shins, **77**
  shoulders, **83**
  sport-specific, 91
  with tennis ball, **80**
  with Thera Cane, 83–84, **89**
  thigh, inner, **89**
Shiatsu, 4, 28, 29
Shin massage
  concentration areas in, 138
  self-massage, **77**
  techniques, **53–55**
Shinsplints, 54
Shorter, Frank, 109, 110, 137
Shoulder massage
  concentration areas in, 138
  self-massage, **83**
  techniques, **39–40**
Skating sports massage techniques, 112–13, **113–15**
Skiing sports massage techniques
  cross-country, 115–16
  downhill, 116, **117–19**
Sleeping, recovery from hard effort and, 128–29, 140
Soles of feet, massaging, **51**
Soleus muscle, 138
Spine massage, **37**, **38**, **41**
Spontaneity in massage, 11–12
Sports massage. *See also* Sports massage techniques
  athletes and
    use of, 1–2, 5
    views of, 151–57

benefits of, 1–2, <u>2</u>, 3, 152
essences for, <u>19</u>
essential oils for, <u>19</u>
feeling effects of, 153–54
as "fourth sport," 154–55
injury prevention and, 1–2, 5, 137–38, 139, 141, 156–57
muscles and, 2–3, <u>2</u>, 29
non-sports massage vs., <u>2</u>
during pregnancy, 156
recovery from hard effort and, 154
regular massage vs., <u>2</u>
relaxation and, 113
therapist, finding or becoming, <u>73</u>
in training, 92
Sports massage techniques, <u>2</u>
    backpacking, 101, **102–3**, 103
    bicycling
        mountain biking, 105, **105–7**
        road, 92, **93–94**, 95
    bodybuilding, 95
    climbing, rock and mountain, 107, **108–9**, 109
    court sports, 95, 96–98, 98
    field sports, 95, **96–98**, 98
    golf, 99–100, **99–100**
    gymnastics, 100–101
    hiking, 101, **102–3**, 103
    kayaking, 103, **104**, 105
    rowing, 103, **104**, 105
    running, 109–10, **110–12**
    self-massage and, 91
    skating, 112–13, **113–15**
    skiing
        cross-country, 115–16
        downhill, 116, **117–19**
    swimming, 119–20, **120–21**
    Thera Cane with, 91
    volleyball, 121–22, **122–23**
    windsurfing, 123, **124–25**
Sport-specific massages. *See* Sports massage techniques
Static stretching, 139
Strengthening exercises
    finger, 7–9, **8**, **9**
    injury prevention and, 92
Stretching
    active, 139
    ballistic, 139
    benefits of, 138–39
    fingers, **8**
    foot, 59
    injury prevention and, 92, 138–39, 141
    massage in combination with, 139, 141
    napping after, <u>140</u>

    passive, 138–39
    proprioreceptive neuromuscular facilitation, 139
    recovery from hard effort and, 139
    static, 139
    toes, **51**, **60**
    in warm-downs, 139
    in warm-ups, 139
Stretching, Inc., 23, 84
Stronglite Massage Table Kits, <u>16</u>
Surfaces, work, for massage, 14–15
Swedish massage, 28
Swedish Movement Treatment, 4
Swelling, cause of, 129
Swimming
    injuries, 119
    sports massage techniques, 119–20, **120–21**

T

Table kit, massage, <u>16</u>
Tables, massage, 14–17
    adjusting, **15**, 17
    with face cradle, 15
    height of, **15**, 17
    kit for building, <u>16</u>
    selecting, 15–16
    self-made, <u>16</u>
    sources for buying, <u>16</u>, 17
Tapotement massage technique, 27, **27**, **28**, 29
Teaford, John, 156–57
Techniques, massage. *See also* Self-massage techniques; Sports massage techniques
    abdomen, 62, **62–64**
    ankles, 49, **49–50**
    arms, 64, **65–69**
    back, 34, **34–41**
    body as guide for, 29–31
    buttocks, 42, **42–43**
    calves, **44**, **47–48**
    chest, 62, **62–64**
    curative/restorative, 32
    deep-tissue, 28, 29, **36**, **45**
    effleurage, 25, **26**, **34**, **44**, **47**, **57**
    exploring different, 11
    face, **71–72**
    feet
        back of, 51, **51–52**
        front of, 59, **59–61**
    friction, 26, **26**, 29, **36**
    hamstrings, 44, **44–48**
    hands, 64, **65–69**
    head, 70, **70–72**

Techniques, massage *(continued)*
  ice, 129–30
  knees, 56, **56**
  legs
    back of, 42, **43**
    front of, 52, **52–53**
  neck, 70, **70–72**
  petrissage, 27, **27**, 29, **41**
  post-event, 32
  pre-event, 32
  quadriceps, **53**, 57, **57–58**
  shiatsu, 28
  shins, **53–55**
  shoulders, **39–40**
  spine, **37**, **38**, **41**
  styles and, basic, 28–29
  Swedish, 28
  tapotement, 27, **27**, **28**, 29
  timing use of, 32, <u>33</u>
  torso
    back of, 34, **34–41**
    front of, 62, **62–64**
  trigger-point therapy, 28
Temperature during massage, body and room, 14
Tendinitis, patellar, 101
Tendons, 42. *See also specific types*
Tennis ball, self-massage with, **80**
Thera Cane, 22
  self-massage with, 83–84, **89**
  sources for buying, 84
  sport-specific massage with, 91
Therapists
  arthritis development in, 10
  breathing of, during massage, 17, 29, 31, **61**
  carpal tunnel syndrome development in, 10
  relaxation of, during massage, 11, 31
  sports massage, finding or becoming, <u>73</u>
Thera Stick, 22
Thigh self-massage, **89**
Thumbsaver, 22
Timing of massage techniques, 32, <u>33</u>
Toes, stretching, **51**, **60**
Tools for massaging
  body tools, 21–23, 83–84
  lubricants, 17–18, <u>19</u>, 20
  music, 20–21
  tables, 14–17

Torso massage techniques
  back of, 34, **34–41**
  front of, 62, **62–64**
Touch, sense of, 3, 23
Toxins, release of body, <u>2</u>, 29, 32, 129
Traction technique, **55**, **60**, **61**, 141
Trager, Milton, <u>149</u>
Trager Institute, <u>149</u>
Trager work, <u>149</u>
Training, sports massage in, 92
Trapezius muscle, 27, **82**
Trenary, Jill, 113
Triathletes, 143–44, 147–48
Triceps, 27, **81**, 123
Trigger-point therapy, 28
Trine, John G., 4

V

Vegetable oils, for massage, 18
Virgin, Craig, 136
Visualization
  during massage, 11
  in mind massage, 146–48
  steps to effective, 147
Volleyball sports massage techniques, 121–22, **122–23**

W

Warm-downs
  napping after, <u>140</u>
  stretching in, 139
Warm-ups, stretching in, 139
Water massage, 10, 131–33, <u>140</u>
Wheat-germ oil, for massage, 18
Windsurfing sports massage techniques, 123, **124–25**
Work surfaces for massage, 14–15

Y

Yarbrough, Carl, 105